**dr foster**

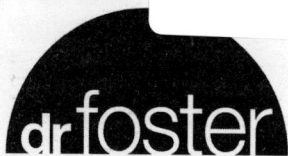

Your Guide to Better Health

# DR FOSTER
# BREAST CANCER
# GUIDE

1 3 5 7 9 10 8 6 4 2

First published 2002 by Vermilion,
an imprint of Ebury Press, Random House,
20 Vauxhall Bridge Road, London SW1V 2SA
www.randomhouse.co.uk

Random House Australia (Pty) Limited
20 Alfred Street, Milsons Point, Sydney,
New South Wales 2061, Australia
Random House New Zealand Limited
18 Poland Road, Glenfield, Auckland 10, New Zealand
Random House South Africa (Pty) Limited
Endulini, 5a Jubilee Road, Parktown 2193, South Africa

The Random House Group Limited Reg. No. 954009

Papers used by Vermilion are natural, recyclable products made from wood grown in sustainable forests.

Printed and bound in Great Britain by
Bookmarque Ltd, Croydon, Surrey

A CIP catalogue record for this book is available
from the British Library

ISBN 0091883822

**dr foster**

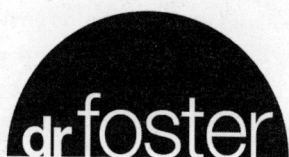

Your Guide to Better Health

# DR FOSTER
# BREAST CANCER
# GUIDE

Researched and Compiled
by Dr Foster
Text by Patsy Westcott

**Vermilion**
LONDON

# Who is Dr Foster?

Dr Foster provides authoritative information on health services of all kinds in the UK. Our aim is to empower patients with information to help them access the best possible care. We are supervised by an independent Ethics committee that has legal powers to ensure that guides meet the highest standards and to investigate complaints.

The Ethics committee currently comprises the following membership:

**Dr Jack Tinker**, dean of the Royal Society of Medicine and chair of the committee

**Sir Donald Irvine**, past president, General Medical Council

**Dr Michael Dixon**, chair, NHS Alliance

**Peter Griffiths**, chief executive, Health Quality Service

**Dianne Hayter**, member of the board of the National Patient Safety Agency and the National Consumer Council

**Professor Alan Maynard**, director, Health Policy Unit, York University and chair, York Health Services NHS Trust

**Wilma MacPherson**, visiting professor at King's College London and a consultant in Health Services

**Bridget Gill**, chair of the Northern and Yorkshire Regional Council of the Institute of Healthcare Management

**Trevor Campbell Davis**, chief executive, Whittington Hospital

**Douglas Webb**, operations and development director, Friends of the Elderly

**Vanessa Bourne**, chair, Patients Association

**Dr Philip Davies**, medical director, Pontypridd and Rhondda NHS Trust

**Professor Nairn Wilson**, president of the General Dental Council.

---

## Dr Foster Help at Hand

Dr Foster collects data on local hospital, maternity and fertility services. It also has comprehensive information on hospital doctors and complementary therapists. Call the

**Help at Hand Service** on **0906 190 0212**

to find the right solution to your health needs.

You can also visit

**www.drfoster.co.uk**

for information.

Calls cost £1.50 per minute; costs from mobile phones and some other networks may be more. Callers must be aged 18 or over. Lines are open Mon to Fri from 8.30am – 8pm, Sat 8.30am – 6pm.

Dr Foster Ltd.
Sir John Lyon House
5 High Timber Street
London EC4V 3NX

---

# Contents

# Acknowledgements

Dr Foster would like to thank the following organisations and individuals for their time and help in compiling the information in this book (they are not, however, in any way responsible for anything included or omitted).

**Breast Cancer Care** is the leading provider of breast cancer information and support in the UK. They provide free services for everyone affected by breast cancer including a helpline, website, publications, and practical and emotional support.

**Christine Fogg** is the Chief Executive of Breast Cancer Care. She initially trained as a nurse, specialising in oncology and haematology and later moved into NHS management within the HIV/AIDS and sexual health field. Prior to working at Breast Cancer Care, Christine was the Chief Executive of two HIV/AIDS charities.

**Dame Gill Oliver** is Director of Service Development for Macmillan Cancer Relief. After starting her career nursing cancer patients, Gill became Director of Patient Services at the Clatterbridge Centre for Oncology in 1992 and joined Macmillan Cancer Relief as Director of Service Development in April 2000. She was a member of the Expert Advisory Group on Cancer that produced the *Calman Hine Report*, and belongs to other national and regional policy and strategy groups.

**Julietta Patnick** is the National Coordinator of the NHS Cancer Screening Programmes. As national coordinator her main interest is in quality assurance, but she is also extensively involved in policy issues, promotion of the programme, developing materials for informed choice and management of the information systems. Mrs Patnick has also worked internationally on cancer screening issues, and has worked on breast screening from the inception and planning stages of the NHSBSP in 1987.

We would also like to thank **Andrea Pearson** at the National Screening office for her help and guidance during compilation of the screening unit surveys, and the Regional Co-ordinators at the Quality Assurance Reference Centres for their assistance in compiling breast screening data.

**Claire Rayner OBE** is a journalist, novelist and broadcaster (both on radio and television). As a trained nurse and midwife, she is an acknowledged authority on child care, medical and allied subjects, but has a special interest in breast cancer, having been a patient herself.

**UK Breast Cancer Coalition** was founded in 1995 by women with personal experience of breast cancer and is the leading UK organisation dedicated to improving breast cancer services through patient advocacy.

**Patsy Westcott** is a writer and journalist. She regularly contributes to the national press, has written over 20 books on health and contributed to several health encyclopaedias and part-works.

We would also like to thank the following consultants for their assistance:

**Professor Steven Heys** (Aberdeen Royal Infirmary)

**Professor David Sharpe** (Bradford Royal Infirmary)

**Mr John N Fox** (Castle Hill Hospital)

**Mr Dudley Sinnett** (Charing Cross Hospital)

**Professor Ian Fentiman** and **Professor Robert Rubens** (Guy's and St Thomas' Hospital)

**Professor Roger Blamey** and **Dr Robin Wilson** (Nottingham City Hospital)

**Professor Mike Baum** (Portland Hospital)

**Dr Alison Jones** (Royal Free Hospital)

**Mr Gerald Gui**, **Professor John Yarnold**, **Mr Nigel Sacks**, **Professor Ian E Smith**, **Dr Stephen Johnston** and **Professor Mitch Dowsett** (Royal Marsden Hospital)

**Professor T W J Lennard** (Royal Victoria Infirmary, Newcastle)

**Dr Kate Gregory** (Southampton General Hospital)

**Mr Robert Carpenter** (St Bartholomew's Hospital)

**Mr Mike Dixon** (Western General Hospital, Edinburgh)

# Foreword by Claire Rayner

Why are you reading this? You certainly didn't pick it up in search of a jolly book to doze over on your holidays. The obvious reason is that you or someone about whom you care deeply has been diagnosed as having breast cancer, and you're looking for information.

When I was diagnosed with breast cancer one breezy May afternoon in 2001, I thought at first, as one who has worked professionally in the medical world for almost fifty years, I wouldn't need much more information than I already had.

I soon realised that there was much I wanted to know. Facts change over the years and news about quality provision changes almost week by week. There have been huge strides forward in the treatment of breast cancer over the last decade and more people than ever before are recovering fully.

What I needed, I decided, was a single volume that would provide all the facts I might want, calm any irrational fears that may have seized me (and believe me, they do from all directions! I know from miserable personal experience just how irrational and fearful the word 'cancer' can make even the most sensible person), and which would generally help me feel that I had at least some control over what was happening to me.

If you are in that situation now, then, pilgrim, your search is ended. In these pages you will find a wealth of answers to your questions. There is a clear account of what cancer is; not just one disease, as so many think, but a multitude of different diseases, all behaving according to their site and the stimuli they might be given.

You will also find answers to questions about breast cancer specifically and possible treatments (including hormone therapy) together with their pros and their cons. You can find out about 'complementary' therapies (non-orthodox methods of care) and balance their uses and risks for you or your special patient.

Of course I may be wrong and you, my new reader, are interested in this book not for personal reasons but for purely professional ones. If you are, or work with, a GP there is as much meat for you in these pages as for your patients. Many of those who come through your doors will come bearing piles of luggage made up of fears, many of them irrational, some all too reasonable but unnecessarily inflated, and some downright myths.

You will find here all the myth-breakers you need and possibly one or two that will get rid of misapprehensions of your own that you might not yet have realised you nurtured.

And there are others who will find in these pages much to think about. Those who are responsible for running our NHS Trusts and Cancer Services in general must surely be deeply concerned, because this Guide, in what is fast becoming the trademark Dr Foster style, includes an exhaustive amount of data about the provision and use of quality care in both the NHS and the Private Sector.

In addition and of great interest to us all, the Guide offers the rates of success of various screening units and five-year survival rates as collected by the country's various Health Authorities.

The facts a newly diagnosed patient, her family and friends need can be found here. What she won't find, of course, is the human ear and the human response that is much more comforting and reassuring than even the best of books can be. The Guide provides information about the many support groups there are for people with cancer, a term which of course includes all the relatives and friends of patients, as well as the patients themselves.

One small warning; remember that the services provided by hospitals and doctors are constantly changing. This book tells you about services in your area but always check details with your GP or other healthcare professionals looking after you.

Use the Guide thoroughly, ask everyone you come across professionally every question you want to, and remember there are an amazing number of people living full rich lives with their cancer who are symptom free and who have every chance of remaining so for many years to come. A diagnosis of cancer is not necessarily the end of anyone's road!

# Understanding breast cancer

# Introduction by Christine Fogg

In the UK almost 40,000 women are diagnosed with breast cancer every year, making it the most common form of cancer in women. That means that each year 40,000 women – and about 250 men – have their lives turned upside down in the most unimaginable way. And of course it doesn't stop there because the impact of that diagnosis extends to their families, friends and colleagues.

At the same time advances in screening and in treatment have resulted in more early diagnosis of breast cancer and better outcomes overall. The UK now has the fastest falling breast cancer mortality rate in the world. This is excellent news. But the fact remains that coming to terms with a diagnosis of breast cancer and what that might mean – while at the same time having to deal with complicated treatment decisions – can often leave people feeling frightened, overwhelmed and powerless.

Breast cancer is a bewildering and complex experience. That's why it is so important that people affected by breast cancer have access to clear, complete and reliable information about services, treatments –and the people involved in providing those treatments. People need information in order to help them make informed decisions and to ensure that they get access to the best treatment available. That's why this guide is such an important step forward.

At Breast Cancer Care we have contact with over 500,000 people a year who are affected by breast cancer in some way. Our experience is that many of those people are seeking support and information, including information about their treatment options, what these options might involve and how breast cancer services in the NHS and the private healthcare sector are structured. Until now this information hasn't been readily available in this kind of format.

This guide is unique and important. It is specifically designed for use within the UK's health system. It explains how cancer services are arranged across the country, what you should do if you're not happy with any aspect of your treatment, as well as the questions you should be asking at every stage. The guide outlines current treatments, covering chemotherapy and availability of drugs, radiotherapy, endocrine therapy surgery, and reconstruction – as well as the importance of financial and emotional support. It also provides information for women who have been diagnosed with secondary breast cancer. Women who we know from our work at Breast Cancer Care can feel especially isolated.

This guide provides comprehensive, up-to-date information about breast cancer and will go a long way to fill the information gap that currently exists for people affected by breast cancer.

# How to use this guide

This guide tells you how breast cancer services are delivered throughout the UK and what different breast units do. The idea is that by combining the two, you can get the best care available in your region.

The book is divided into two sections. The first outlines treatments you might have and asks questions about services, like the ones above. We also have stories by both patients and those in charge of care to give you an idea of what might be expected depending on your diagnosis and region.

The second section gives you information on specific breast units, private and NHS. For each NHS clinic we list the volumes and waiting times for mastectomies and lumpectomies, details of patient information provided, names of breast surgeons and the location and type of treatment for which you may be referred elsewhere. Information is also provided on breast screening units, including the interval between invitations for screening and cancer detection rates for each unit. For private clinics we tell you where they are, whether they have a BUPA-approved breast unit, whether they provide radiotherapy, chemotherapy and palliative care and which insurers will pay for treatment there.

The Guide aims to be as comprehensive as possible in its listing of treatments and support available. Whatever your diagnosis and wherever you live, the Dr Foster Breast Cancer Guide tells you everything you need to know to get the best treatment and support possible. For example:

**How is breast cancer care organised in my area?**
On page 133 we explain how cancer services are arranged in Cancer Networks and how this influences the way your treatment is provided.

**I don't want to go to the hospital I have been referred to. Can I attend a different hospital for my tests?**
The creation of Cancer Networks (see p.133) means that the facilities in different areas should offer the same standard of service throughout the country. If for some reason you don't want to attend

the hospital your GP has referred you to, you should discuss it with them, explaining your reasons. On page 26 we explain what you can expect in this situation.

**How long am I likely to have to wait between seeing my GP and being seen by a specialist?**

Waiting times are one of the biggest issues in the NHS today, particularly with the Government's introduction of cancer waiting time targets. Under the NHS National Cancer Plan, anyone with suspected cancer should be able to see a specialist within two weeks of being urgently referred by their GP. On page 26 we give you an idea of what this is likely to mean for you.

# Understanding breast cancer

Cancer is an uncontrolled growth and proliferation of cells, with the potential to invade surrounding tissue and to spread to other parts of the body. There are many different kinds of cancer, affecting different organ systems. The causes, the underlying process by which it develops, the symptoms, the response to treatment and the long-term outlook vary with each cancer type. However, each cancer begins in the same way: with the uncontrolled division of a single cell.

Throughout our lives our body's cells are constantly dividing and reproducing (replicating). This enables damaged cells to be repaired and old cells to be replaced. The process of repair and maintenance is regulated by genes, which instruct the cells to begin dividing and tell them when to stop. Normally the whole process happens in a controlled way. However, sometimes a mutant gene causes a fault to occur in the cell. Cells within our body tissue make such errors from time to time but these don't always cause a cancerous change. The body has a series of biological checkpoints at which damaged cells can be stalled to prevent them developing into cancer. However, especially as we get older and our bodies become less efficient, a damaged cell sometimes evades the natural checking mechanism and carries on replicating. Eventually, the cluster of cells becomes so large that it forms a mass. Depending on which part of your body is affected, it may be visible or felt (palpable) as a lump or tumour.

The development of a faulty cell into a tumour is a relatively long, slow process. In fact most adult cancers, including breast cancer, may take years to develop. Tumours can be benign (non-cancerous) or malignant (cancerous).

- **Benign tumours.** These remain confined to a particular organ or tissue and do not spread or threaten life.
- **Malignant tumours.** The key characteristic of cancer cells is that, unless halted, they are capable of invading and destroying surrounding tissues. They may then migrate into the bloodstream or lymphatic system to form secondary tumours elsewhere in the body, a process known as metastasis.

**What is breast cancer and are all breast cancers the same?**

Like all cancers, breast cancer happens when the cells of the breast replicate uncontrollably. There are several different types, each of which has different symptoms, different patterns of progress and a different long-term outlook. For further details on the different types see page 39.

**Who is at risk?**

All women are at risk of developing breast cancer. A small number of men also develop breast cancer (see p.9). In the UK, your chance of developing breast cancer at some time if you reach the age of 85 is around one in 10. Although this may sound rather alarming, the high figure partly reflects the fact that doctors have become better at detecting cancer at an early stage, and that most of these cancers will occur in women over the age of 60; breast cancer in young women is rare. The good news is that, thanks to earlier diagnosis and better treatments, fewer women are dying of breast cancer.

Certain factors increase your risk of developing breast cancer. These include:

- **Previous breast cancer.** This increases your risk of developing it in your other breast, although the increase is only 1 per cent per year.
- **Benign breast disease in the past for which you have had a biopsy.** Certain non-cancerous conditions and atypical hyperplasia (overgrowth of the breast cells) can increase your risk.
- **Exposure to radiation while young.** If your breasts were exposed to radiation (for example, by having radiotherapy for another cancer such as Hodgkin's disease), your risk of developing breast cancer is increased.
- **Your genetic inheritance.** Your risk of developing breast cancer increases if your mother, sister or daughter had the disease, especially at a young age (see p.16). However, it is important to remember that only 5–10 per cent of patients appear to be affected by genetic inheritance.
- **An early start to periods and/or late menopause.** Starting to menstruate before the age of 12 and having the menopause after 55 increases your risk.
- **Never having children.** Women who have never had children are at a higher risk.

- **Having children over the age of 30.** Research shows that having a first child after the age of 30 pushes up your risk.
- **Not breastfeeding long term.** Women who breastfeed for long periods, especially their first child, appear to have a lower risk. This may be because it causes hormonal changes, such as decreasing the level of oestrogen and suppressing ovulation. According to some studies, women who have fewer ovulatory cycles over the course of their reproductive lives may have a reduced risk. Breastfeeding may also cause physical changes in the cells that line the mammary ducts, making them more resistant to mutations that can lead to cancer.
- **Use of oral contraception or HRT.** There are controversial findings that suggest that prolonged use of the Pill or HRT may cause a slightly increased risk while you are taking the therapy, although this decreases once you have stopped. (See p.13.)
- **Being overweight.** Post-menopausal women who are 40 per cent over their ideal body weight are at greater risk of developing breast cancer, although it is not yet known exactly why. One theory is that, after the menopause, oestrogen is converted in its active form in the body fat, with the result that there is more circulating oestrogen in the bloodstream. Another is that toxins in fatty tissue may be released into the bloodstream and damage breast cells.
- **Alcohol intake.** The possible role of alcohol in the development of breast cancer is controversial. An increasing number of studies suggest that regularly drinking alcohol can increase your risk. Research carried out at the Harvard School of Public Health, USA, found that four or five alcoholic drinks a day can push up the risk of breast cancer by 41 per cent. However, other research studies have not found an association. Some experts believe that alcohol may only increase the risk of breast cancer when combined with another risk factor such as taking HRT.

### Can men get breast cancer?

Yes, although male cases account for less than one per cent of breast cancers. The condition is most often diagnosed between the ages of 60 and 70. Risk factors include exposure to radiation, high levels of oestrogen in the body (caused, for example, by liver disease or

# Val Day

I had a routine mammogram, and a month after having that I was asked to go back to Bart's Hospital and was diagnosed in June 2001. Telling the children was really difficult as that particular weekend when I found out about it was our Ruby Wedding Anniversary, so the children were here with their partners. We kept it quiet until about ten days later when not telling them became a burden.

I had to wait just four and a bit weeks between the final diagnosis and the op and then I had a lumpectomy. They found a second lump behind the one they knew about and took that away, and they took lymph nodes from the armpit to check out.

There are a lot of 'mights' in it: this might happen, that might happen, but I must say I had covered all the scariest things because I'd had experience with my daughter, Nicola, who was diagnosed when she was 33. She found a tiny pea-sized lump during a self-examination in October 2000, went to the GP, was referred straight away to the hospital and had a lumpectomy in November. And then she was asked to go in again for some tests, and when she went for her results she was told that they had discovered pre-cancerous cells in the breast, and they recommended a mastectomy. That was an awful blow, a bad day. The op was done in January 2001.

She had fantastic care in Nottingham at the City Hospital. She had a young breast cancer nurse who was absolutely totally genned up and very, very supportive and took her through the whole thing. I met her when I went to Nottingham for Nic's implant operation, which they did in July, just a week before mine. So I didn't have a lot of time really to worry about myself because I focused on her right up until the day I came back from Nottingham, and the following day I went into hospital. Maybe that was naïve, but it got me through.

The one piece of information I didn't get until afterwards was the seriousness of the lump. I assumed that because Nicola's surgery was bigger, that her's was worse. It turned out that hers was a grade 1 and mine was a grade 3. I didn't think to ask at the time, and it probably saved me a lot of worry, but that information was not volunteered.

Nicola went down every possible avenue that was offered to her: diet and complementary medicines, everything that was a possible factor she investigated. I didn't, simply because I didn't feel I needed to: I knew the nitty gritty, and as far as I was concerned the advice and the treatment that I had was enough; I didn't look elsewhere at all. Friends and family were of course wonderfully supportive.

I don't think there is a family connection to our breast cancers. I've discussed it with the doctors I've been under, and there was an option for us to look into the possible heredity factor, but my daughter wasn't keen to go into that side of things. There's no history of it anywhere else in the family at all, and we've just come to the conclusion that it's an unhappy coincidence that she got it and I got it as well. I might have wished it on myself by thinking when she told me she had it: 'Why not me?' So, who knows?

certain genetic disorders such as Klinefelter's syndrome) and a family history of breast cancer, especially where the family members affected have a mutation of one of the breast cancer genes.

## Is male breast cancer different to female breast cancer?

Doctors used to think that male breast cancer was different to female cancer, due to the fact that although fewer men developed it, a higher percentage died from it. It is now known that this is not the case. The most common type is ductal cancer. Inflammatory Breast Cancer and Paget's Disease of the nipple can also affect men. If diagnosed relatively early, the outlook for men is similar to that of women. Their apparently poorer outlook is thought to be a result of the fact that men tend to be diagnosed at a later stage.

## At what age am I most at risk of developing breast cancer?

Like many cancers, breast cancer usually takes a long time to develop so the risk increases with age. Just 2 per cent of breast cancers affect women under 35 while some 40 per cent are detected in the over 70s. Because breast cells are less active as we get older, such cancers usually develop very slowly. The most common age to be diagnosed is around 50. Below shows the increasing risk with age:

| Your age | Your risk |
| --- | --- |
| 15–25 | One in 15,000 |
| 26–30 | One in 1,900 |
| 31–40 | One in 200 |
| 41–50 | One in 50 |
| 51–60 | One in 23 |
| 61–70 | One in 15 |
| 71–80 | One in 11 |
| 81–85 | One in 10 |

## How are hormones involved in breast cancer?

Exposure to the female sex hormone oestrogen is closely related to the risk of developing breast cancer. The more oestrogen you are exposed to during the course of your lifetime – either that produced by your own body (endogenous) or from drugs or other sources (exogenous) – the greater your risk of breast cancer. One of the actions of oestrogen is to cause breast cells to multiply and develop during each menstrual cycle in preparation for a potential pregnancy. When breast cells are active in this way, they are more prone to develop errors that could grow into cancer.

## Could being on the Pill have increased my risk?

The oral contraceptive Pill does slightly increase the risk of developing breast cancer, although the relative risk is small. Doctors would expect to diagnose only one extra case of breast cancer for every 20,000 women using the Pill between the ages of 20 and 25. The risk is only raised as long as you take the Pill. Once you stop taking it, your risk gradually reduces and disappears completely when you have stopped taking it for ten years. Incidentally, breast cancer tends to be diagnosed earlier in women taking the Pill, suggesting perhaps that these women are more conscious of their reproductive health and may therefore check their breasts more often.

If you have an inherited predisposition to develop breast cancer (see p.16), there is research suggesting that your risk of developing the disease may be greater if you take the Pill, although it also protects against the risk of ovarian cancer, which is raised in some women with inherited breast cancer genes. If you have a family history of breast cancer, you should seek medical advice about the most appropriate form of contraception.

## What about Hormone Replacement Therapy (HRT)?

The picture is rather muddier when it comes to HRT and studies have been contradictory. It is generally agreed that taking HRT for five years or longer slightly increases your risk of developing breast cancer, although the risk returns to normal when you stop taking HRT. Research from the US suggests that the risk is higher in women taking combined HRT (that is, oestrogen and progesterone) than in women on unopposed HRT (oestrogen alone), though data remains controversial. On the other hand, research also shows that women on HRT diagnosed with breast cancer are less likely to die of the disease than women who have not taken HRT. There may be many reasons for this, including the fact that women taking HRT may be more health-conscious generally and are also likely to be having regular medical check-ups so any cancer is likely to be diagnosed at an early stage. For more on HRT and breast cancer, see page 99. It is up to you to weigh up the relative benefits and risks of HRT for you personally in discussion with your doctor.

## How can I reduce my risk?

The prevention of any illness consists of avoiding known risk factors where possible and increasing any factors that may protect you so your chance of developing the condition decreases. In the case of breast cancer, this means making an effort to understand how the risk factors listed may apply to you personally and trying to modify them by making healthy choices. The following measures will benefit your health and sense of well-being generally and may help protect you against other diseases such as heart disease, diabetes and other forms of cancer.

**Watch what you eat:** Diet is thought to play a contributory role in 30 to 40 per cent of all cancers and rates of breast cancer are lowest in countries where people's diet is made up mostly of plant-based foods, fruit, vegetables, oily fish, unsaturated fats, nuts and seeds. Eating healthily cannot insure you completely against breast cancer, but it may help reduce your chance of developing it and it is beneficial for your heart, bones and immune system.

- Eat more fruit and vegetables (aim for five portions a day).
- Cut down on meat and animal fat: US research suggests that reducing fat intake dramatically can reduce oestrogen levels and so potentially lower the risk of developing breast cancer, although the long-running US Nurses' Health Study revealed no evidence that lowering fat intake or changing the kinds of fat women ate affected their breast cancer risk. It could be that a diet high in fat increases the risk of obesity, which is a known risk factor, rather than fat in itself.

**Moderate your alcohol intake:** The American Cancer Society now suggests limiting alcohol intake to one unit a day or giving it up altogether, although British cancer charities have not yet gone this far.

- Aim to keep your alcohol intake to one unit a day or give up altogether, especially if you have a number of other risk factors.
- If you do drink, make sure you eat plenty of fruit and vegetables. Research from the Nurses' Health Study found that women who had a high intake of folic acid (found in green leafy veg, such as

spinach, kale and broccoli, apricots, fortified cereals) may protect themselves from breast cancer when they drink alcohol.

**Take regular exercise:** A growing number of studies suggests that being physically active may help to reduce the risk of breast cancer, although it is not known what kind of exercise is most beneficial, which women benefit most, how much activity is needed or at what stage in life it is most beneficial. It is also not known whether it is exercise itself or its effect on weight which is the key factor.

**Stay breast aware:** Get to know how your breasts look and feel normally. That way you should be able to detect any changes and report them to your doctor, bearing in mind that nine out of 10 breast lumps are not cancerous.

**Look after your reproductive health:** Make informed choices about contraception and HRT. Once you reach the age of 50, take advantage of the NHS National Screening Programme (see p.22).

**Know your genetic risk:** If there is a history of breast cancer in your family (see p.16 for details), it is a good idea to get your GP to refer you to a family history clinic to find out what measures you can take that may help reduce your risk. It is important to understand that strategies for risk reduction are still developing, and there is a lot of uncertainty about risk reduction measures.

### Is there any way to guarantee I won't get breast cancer?

Until more is known about the exact causes of breast cancer, there is nothing you can do to insure yourself against it completely. Even avoiding risk factors is no guarantee, although it can help you feel more in control of your body and may help to reduce your odds. It is worth bearing in mind that most people with a particular risk factor – even those with a strong genetic susceptibility – will not get the disease.

### I've heard that eating a diet high in plant oestrogens can help protect against breast cancer. Is this true?

A great deal is written in books and magazines about the potential role of diet in breast cancer. One of the most popular stories is that soya foods and other fruit, vegetables and seeds (such as lentils, chickpeas, flax seeds and the herb red clover) containing phyto-oestrogens (weak plant oestrogens that mimic the action of the female sex hormone) may reduce the risk of breast cancer. Some studies have shown that Japanese women whose diets are high in soya have a far lower incidence of breast cancer than women in the West. When these women move to the West and eat a typical Western diet their breast cancer risk rises.

Although the results look promising, scientists have still not worked out exactly how soya and other phyto-oestrogens might act, and some important questions remain unanswered. It is difficult to determine whether the Japanese women's advantage stems from the fact that they have consumed a diet high in soya all their lives and exactly how much soya is needed to have a protective effect.

The picture is even more complicated when it comes to women with breast cancer. Doctors are concerned that soya may compete with tamoxifen, a hormonal treatment that is often prescribed for women with breast cancer. There are also fears that a high soy diet may actually encourage the progression of certain kinds of breast cancer that are fuelled by oestrogen.

**My mother had breast cancer. Am I likely to develop it?**
That depends on the type of breast cancer she had, when she developed it and whether any other close relatives (for example, your maternal grandmother or aunts, your sister or daughter) have also been affected. Because breast cancer is common, many of us will have relatives who have had the disease without having an abnormal gene. In most cases there is no need for you to worry. If your mother developed cancer after the age of 55, your increased risk is small. However, in a small number of cases – between 5 and 10 per cent – breast cancer is caused by a single mutant gene that is passed down through the family. So far, two breast cancer genes, BRCA1 and BRCA2, have been identified and other genes such as P53 – which is responsible for controlling cell growth throughout the body – are also known to be involved.

Both men and women can carry the BRCA genes, which are also linked to other forms of cancer, most notably ovarian, but also pancreatic, stomach, bowel and (in men) prostate cancer. If you have one of these genes you have a one-in-two lifetime risk of developing breast cancer, although you are by no means certain to develop it.

## How can I find out if I have inherited a faulty gene?

Short of having a gene test (see below), you can't know for sure. However, there are certain patterns that suggest you may be at risk. These include:

- First-degree female relative (i.e. mother, sister, daughter) with breast cancer diagnosed below the age of 40.
- Two first- or second-degree female relatives (i.e. aunt, cousin, grandmother) with breast cancer diagnosed below the age of 60, or ovarian cancer at any age.
- A first- or second-degree female relative with breast and ovarian cancer diagnosed at any age.
- Three first- or second-degree female relatives with breast or ovarian cancer at any age.
- A first-degree female relative who has developed cancer in both breasts (bilateral cancer) with the first breast cancer developing below the age of 60.
- A first-degree male relative with breast cancer at any age.

## What should I do if I suspect there is an inherited risk of breast cancer in my family?

Consult your GP, who may refer you to a family cancer clinic. Here they will try to assess your risk, and may offer you regular screening plus advice on measures to reduce your risk and ensure that any cancer you may develop is diagnosed as early as possible. Hopefully, once more research has been done, more effective risk reduction methods will be found.

## Should I have a gene test?

In some cases, where there is a member or members of the living family who have been diagnosed with breast cancer, it is possible to have a blood test to check whether your DNA has a faulty gene. This is not an easy decision to make. There is the thorny problem of how you will deal with the information should you discover that you do possess one of the faulty breast cancer genes. The very last thing anyone wants is to spend the rest of their life paralysed with fear. Even if you do have a faulty gene, no one can tell you if or when you might develop breast cancer. Studies of identical twins, for example, both of whom have a breast cancer gene, have shown that it is by no means certain that if one develops the disease the other will do so too, although research has shown that it is more likely than for non-identical twins who do not share the same gene.

**Pros and cons of genetic testing**

**Pros**

- You will know whether you are genetically predisposed to develop breast cancer.
- This could help you make decisions about your lifestyle and other measures. For example, whether to consider having a prophylactic mastectomy (see below).
- If the test is negative, you are likely to feel tremendously relieved – both for yourself and any daughters you may have.

**Cons**

- If a gene or genes are found, you have the worry of knowing for certain that you have a genetic susceptibility to develop breast cancer.
- Danger of complacency if you discover there is no genetic risk. A negative gene test doesn't mean you will never develop the disease.
- As it is early days for genetic screening and risk reduction having a genetic test might cause a lot of unnecessary anxiety.

**Can I still have a gene test if I don't have a family history?**

With the exception of the above instances, breast cancer is rarely caused by a single gene. It is more often the result of the cumulative action of several common genes that many of us carry, each of which slightly raises the overall risk. Currently, predictions of breast cancer risk are not very accurate. However, as more and more genes predisposing us to it are found, this is likely to change. In a report published in *Nature Genetics* (March 2002), scientists revealed that over half of all breast cancers are likely to occur in just 12 per cent of women carrying a combination of these genes. In future, rather than screening everyone, it may be possible to specifically identify women at high risk by testing for a selection of these genes. It is thought that this will be far more effective than current methods of prediction based on risk factors. However, such mass genetic screening is still some way in the future.

**If I have a high genetic risk of breast cancer, could having my breasts removed prevent me developing it?**

Some women with a higher risk of developing breast cancer decide to have their breasts removed (a prophylactic mastectomy) to try to reduce their risk. Two recent studies have shown how effective this is:

- The US Mayo Clinic looked at sisters who were at high risk of inherited breast cancer. They found that mastectomy reduced the risk of developing the disease by around 90 per cent and also reduced the number of women dying.

- A second study, in the Netherlands, compared 139 women who were carrying BRCA1/2 mutations, half of whom chose regular surveillance and half of whom chose prophylactic mastectomy. At the end of two years, eight breast cancers had been diagnosed in the surveillance group and none among those who chose prophylactic mastectomy.

Prophylactic mastectomy is a drastic option that not all women with a genetic risk will feel is right for them. What we do now know is that it is a viable option if you have a high risk of developing breast cancer.

**Pros and cons**

**Pros**

- Substantial reduction of risk of breast cancer and the sense of relief this can bring.

**Cons**

- Subjecting yourself to the risks of major surgery – both mastectomy and reconstruction if you opt for this – when you are not actually ill.

- No guarantee you will avoid breast cancer. Breast tissue is not confined to the breasts. It extends up to the collarbone, down to the abdominal wall and under the armpits. Given this widespread distribution, it is virtually impossible for a surgeon to remove every last breast cell.

**Are there drugs that can stop me getting breast cancer if I have a family history?**

Chemoprevention is the use of drugs to prevent cancer. The most well-known chemopreventive is tamoxifen, a drug that works by blocking the action of oestrogen on breast cells, preventing cancer

# Joan Bartram

I started off with a lump in my breast about ten years ago. I had it removed, but then three years ago a lump appeared in exactly the same place, so I had to lose my breast.

When I was treated for the first lump I had radiotherapy and tamoxifen, and of course after five years I was discharged. They told me to come in for a check-up mammogram and that was when they found the second lump. The surgeon said I couldn't have radiotherapy or tamoxifen again. He said that one of my choices was to join a trial they were running for some new drugs. In a way I had no choice really; I'd been through the other things and I was hoping I wouldn't have to have chemotherapy, which was the only thing I hadn't had, so when he suggested joining the trial I thought why not? I didn't hesitate; I knew it might not work, or that it might make me very ill, but I thought: 'it might help others as well, what have I got to lose? Let's have a go and see what happens' so I went ahead.

I suppose I was a little bit nervous about being on a trial; after all, when it's a trial there is an idea that you don't know what's going to happen, really. I was a little worried - I mean, no one else had even heard of what I was on, but there was never any pressure to be on the trial. I suppose I am a bit like a guinea-pig in some ways! Even now when I get a prescription, the chemist has to order it in specially!

The trial was for Femara and Arimidex, and I have to say, I didn't know an awful lot about it. I was just told that it was two different drugs. I had to try two tablets after my last operation, the first for a certain amount of time, then a break and then the second tablet. The first, Arimidex,  didn't suit me at all: I felt awful, nauseous and ill. I had to write down every day what I felt (awful) and how my family felt about what I was doing, although they were very agreeable to the whole thing. I stopped taking the first tablet then had to wait two weeks to see what would happen. I started to feel well again, but I thought: 'if this doesn't work, what is the next step? ' Luckily I had no after-effects on Femara at all.

I'm glad I took part in the trial; I just hope that other women can benefit in the way I did; I had such awful side-effects on the other drug, finding an alternative was wonderful.

cells from growing and dividing in some kinds of breast cancer. This drug is not currently licensed for preventative use in the UK as, although there is evidence that tamoxifen can prevent breast cancer from recurring in women who have been treated for the disease and that it can also prevent cancer from spreading (metastasis), it is still not known whether it can prevent breast cancer in high-risk women who do not have the disease. In one large trial, the drug reduced the risk of invasive breast cancer in a group of such women by 49 per cent. However, studies have also shown that tamoxifen does not completely eliminate the risk of developing breast cancer. Research continues, and it will be some time before there are definitive answers. Doctors are also investigating other chemopreventive drugs such as anastrozole and raloxifene, which block the effects of oestrogen and may have fewer side-effects than tamoxifen.

### Can I ask to have a mammogram even if I don't have any symptoms of breast cancer?

You won't usually be able to have a mammogram on the NHS until you reach 50, unless you have symptoms. If you have private medical insurance or belong to a private health plan that includes Well Woman Screening, you may be offered a mammogram and/or ultrasound as part of that, although it is important to bear in mind that ultrasound should not be regarded as an alternative to mammography. However, if you are under 50, mammograms are less efficient at picking up changes because the breast tissue of younger women is denser and more difficult to X-ray. The best way to ensure any breast cancer is picked up early is to learn to be breast aware, becoming familiar with what is normal for you, so that you are aware of any changes. Learning how your breasts feel at different times will help you know what is normal for you. For example, some women's breasts become lumpy pre-menstrually. Knowing this might help you identify something that should be checked by your doctor.

### When will I be eligible for the NHS breast screening programme?

All women aged between 50 and 64 are eligible to have a mammogram at least every three years. The exact interval between mammograms varies throughout the country. Older women can continue to have mammograms on request, and by 2004 the national programme will be extended to include women aged 65 to 70. If the mammogram shows no signs of cancer, you will be invited to return in another three years. If the mammogram reveals early signs of breast cancer or is unclear, you will be referred to a breast unit for further assessment (see p.25).

**How will I be invited to be screened?**
Provided you are registered with a GP, you will be sent an appointment through the post within three years of your fiftieth birthday inviting you to attend a local screening centre.

# Detection and diagnosis

Women find most breast cancers themselves. Each woman's breasts are different in shape, size and texture and they change throughout life. As you grow older, for example, they become softer and less lumpy. It is important to become familiar with your own breasts, checking how they look and feel so that you know what is normal for you. If you find anything unusual, you will be in a better position to work out whether what you are seeing or feeling is a part of the normal changes that every woman's breasts go through, or a sign of something that needs investigation. If you do detect anything unusual, try not to panic. Most breast abnormalities are not cancer. Wait and reassess your symptoms after your next period. If the lump is still there or you still have other symptoms, make an appointment with your GP. Changes to watch out for:

- A painless lump or thickened area of tissue in the breast or armpit.
- A change in the shape or size of a breast. For example, one breast is smaller or the breast looks or feels different to usual.
- Enlarged glands under the armpit or swelling of the upper arm.
- Changes in the way the skin of the breast looks (dimpling, puckering or 'tethering' of the skin, a rash, redness or inflammation).
- Change in the nipples. For example, inversion (turning in) of a nipple, discharge from the nipple, rash or swelling on the nipple or area surrounding it (areola) or a lump or thickening of the nipple or the skin surrounding it.

Remember, what you are looking for is a change in what is normal for you.

## Can breast pain be a symptom of cancer?

Breast pain is extremely common, affecting around two out of three women at some stage in their lives. It is also one of the most common reasons for women to be referred to a breast clinic. Although disturbing, pain isn't usually a symptom of breast cancer. In fact many perfectly healthy women have slightly lumpy, tender breasts, especially before their period. Some types of benign (non-cancerous) breast lumps may also be painful. However, pain is the symptom that initially drives some 4–5 per cent of women with breast cancer to seek medical help, although it is not always clear whether the cancer is causing pain or whether a coincidental pain has drawn attention to a cancer.

**What should I do if I have any symptoms?**
The first step is to make an appointment to see your GP. If they think you need further investigation on the grounds of your symptoms, your age or your medical history, they will refer you to a specialist breast clinic for tests. The NHS National Cancer Plan has issued all doctors with guidelines to help them decide when to refer a woman urgently to a breast clinic. Being referred to such a clinic does not mean you have breast cancer. Most women attending for assessment come away with a clean bill of breast health.

**Questions to ask your doctor**

- What are the possible causes of my symptoms?
- Are you referring me to a breast clinic? If so, why? If not, why not?
- Does the hospital you are referring me to have a dedicated breast assessment unit? (see p.41)
- How long am I likely to have to wait for an appointment?
- How will I receive my appointment?
- Can I expect to have my results on the same day?
- If I have to wait for results, how long is this likely to be?
- What should I do if I feel worried while I am waiting for my appointment?

**I had a mammogram under the NHS screening programme and now I've been asked to go to the breast assessment clinic. Does this mean I have breast cancer?**
Since the introduction of the NHS National Screening Service, an increasing number of breast abnormalities are picked up by mammogram before they can be felt or seen. However, if you are recalled for further assessment following a mammogram, it doesn't mean you have breast cancer. In fact, breast cancer is detected in just one in eight women who are referred for further assessment. In some cases, the mammogram is unclear and needs to be repeated. In

others a benign breast problem has been detected that needs investigation. In a small number of cases there may be a cancer or the beginnings of a cancer. The good news is that cancers picked up early in this way can usually be treated extremely effectively.

## How long am I likely to have to wait between seeing my GP and being seen by a specialist?

The period between finding an abnormality and seeing a consultant can be an extremely anxious one and it is natural to want to be seen as quickly as possible. Under the NHS National Cancer Plan, anyone with suspected cancer should be able to see a specialist within two weeks of being urgently referred by their GP. Almost 96 per cent of patients are seen within this time span.

## Can I speed up my appointment?

Most surgeons operate a 'triage system' – that is, they read the referral letters from various GPs in the area and allocate priority to those the GPs think need to be seen most urgently. If there is a real suspicion of breast cancer, most surgeons will see someone faster if contacted by the patient's GP. If you believe you haven't been referred urgently enough, make another appointment with your GP to clarify exactly why they think you don't need an earlier appointment.

## I don't want to go to the hospital I have been referred to. Can I attend a different hospital for my tests?

The creation of Cancer Networks (see p.35) means that the facilities in different areas should offer the same standard of service throughout the country. If for some reason you don't want to attend the hospital your GP has referred you to, you should discuss it with them, explaining your reasons. Your GP may be able to reassure you. If you are still unhappy, you can tell your GP which hospital you wish to be referred to and they should be able to arrange it. However, bear in mind that it may take longer to arrange a referral to a different hospital. You can choose to go privately if you have funds, although it is important to realise that facilities for diagnosis will not necessarily be better than, or indeed as good as, those in an NHS hospital. If you do decide to have private treatment, it is just as important to ask the questions you would ask about NHS treatment.

## What will happen at the breast clinic?

It is natural to feel worried if you have been asked to attend a breast clinic. The staff appreciate how you feel and will do their best to make your visit as stress free as possible. Sometimes you will be sent details of what to expect at your particular clinic when you receive confirmation of your appointment. If you are at all unsure of what to expect and are worried, do not be afraid to call beforehand and ask. Typically an appointment will involve several different stages, although these may vary depending on the unit.

### Arrival

At reception you'll be shown where to wait. It can help to take a book or magazine to read or a friend or relative to talk to in case you have to wait. When it is your turn to be seen, a nurse will call you and take you to a consultation room.

### Taking a history

The doctor or breast care nurse will ask you some questions about your medical history and symptoms. Describe any symptoms as simply, clearly and specifically as you can. The doctor or nurse will make notes and will ask you questions to supplement the information you have given, such as your general health, your reproductive history (whether you have given birth and how many children you have, together with details of any miscarriages, terminations and whether you have taken or are taking the Pill or HRT). You'll also be asked questions specifically relating to your breasts such as whether you have previously had any breast lumps or cysts that may be evidence of benign (non-cancerous) breast disease and whether you or any other members of your family have had breast cancer.

### Clinical examination

You'll then be asked to undress to the waist and the doctor will perform a breast examination. They will look at your breasts and will palpate (feel) them when you are lying down and standing up, paying particular attention to any lumps or swellings. They will also feel under your arms and around the base of your neck for swollen lymph nodes, which could indicate that cancer has spread beyond the breast.

### Tests and procedures

A number of different diagnostic tests and procedures will also be done. The basic three are: mammogram (breast X-ray), an ultrasound scan (which uses sound waves to check for abnormalities) and some

# A GP's perspective

I think being a female GP makes a difference to the way I approach breast cancer, no two ways about it. Not only breast cancer, but any field of female problems. Simple things like PMT, which men can't really understand , even with a sympathetic approach. Really, I think there is a big difference between a male and a female looking at female problems. To realise what a patient is going through when she finds a lump in her breast is so important: I'm pretty sure that most men can't understand the worry, the things going on in a patient's mind.

Generally, I would say that in a month I see about 20 to 30 patients who come here with worries about their breasts. It's education: media, books, papers etc give patients so much information and awareness of the problem that patients become concerned and want to have their breasts examined. Normally we can give them leaflets and things, but some of them are very anxious. If they are having their period, I explain the effects of the hormones on the breasts and I call them back to be examined after their period, after explaining to them the anatomy of the breasts and what happens to the breast tissue. If they belong to an older group, over 30, I examine them straightaway to see what is happening. And you know when you explain to them, so many of them say: 'Oh gosh, half my worry is gone, really.' or 'I'm really feeling relieved.' And you can see the difference. Many of them are satisfied, but then again there are worriers and more problems when there is a family history. No matter how much you explain to them that if at the age of 70 a relative has had breast cancer, even if she's a grandmother it's not too worrying because of her age, the anxiety is still there because they'll have seen her suffer, or have heard from their own mothers how awful it was. I couldn't say no to examining a patient like that, to tell you the truth. Once I have examined her and can see that no matter what I have explained and what leaflets I have given her, the anxiety is still there, then I say: 'That's fair enough,' and the moment I say that OK, we'll organise a mammogram: things improve! You can see the patient's anxiety level dropping down. Out of the 20 or 30 patients I see every month with worries about their breasts I would say that at least 30 to 40 per cent are referred for mammograms, and out of that 30 to 40 per cent I would say that only maybe about 3 or 4 per cent you would say really need to have the mammogram; you are worried, or you kind of suspect something is wrong.

There is the other side, however. We had a patient who had had a lump for about five years, and you didn't really have to examine her. It was just so horrible, really. She's still there, but it was so frightening. When I asked her 'Why did you not come before?' she said, 'Because I was scared'. And again, all the [older] patients of ours, they will come in with a problem and say, 'Oh, so sorry to waste your time.' and I say 'No, really, it's nice to see you, come back!' They feel so obliged for the time you have given or what you tell them. If you have a problem, don't sit at home and think that it will go away. Come here, you know? In our experience, encouraging patients like this does good, because often you catch things just in time.

kind of biopsy. A biopsy will either involve removing a sample of cells for testing, or removing a sliver of tissue, known as a core biopsy. The cells or tissue sample will then be examined under a microscope to check for abnormalities.

You'll find exact details of what these involve below. Depending on the facilities in your area, the various tests may all be done in the breast clinic itself or may involve a visit to a breast screening unit or the hospital's 'imaging' department.

**Receiving results**

Some diagnostic breast clinics offer a 'one stop' service where you can get the results of basic tests such as mammography, breast ultrasonography and fine needle aspiration on the same day. In some units the whole visit, including tests and results, is guaranteed to take just four hours. In some cases, further tests may be needed (see below). Whether they can be done immediately will depend on the facilities available at your particular hospital. If further investigations are needed, most breast care teams will aim to give you your results within seven to 14 days or sooner if possible. The breast unit will also send a letter to your GP containing your diagnosis or probable diagnosis.

Some women would rather have their results on the same day and there are pros and cons to this. One advantage is that you will know one way or another whether you have breast cancer by the time you go home, so there is no anxious waiting period. Other women feel that there are disadvantages to an immediate diagnosis. For example, there may be a lot of waiting around for tests and results on an already stressful day. Also, it can be a bigger shock emotionally, and difficult to take in all at once, although this will depend on your state of mind and the way in which you are treated at the clinic. At any rate, you should be able to discuss the results with a breast care nurse or counsellor. You may also want to take a partner or friend with you to support you.

There are some advantages to having to wait for your results. The waiting time can be a period in which you can prepare yourself mentally and consider your options should you receive a diagnosis of cancer. In addition, your consultant will have had time to prepare a list of treatment options or even a treatment plan for you. Of course, the waiting period can be a time of extreme anxiety and mixed emotions, but in many units you will be given a dedicated phone number to call where you can discuss any questions and anxieties with a specialist breast care nurse. If this is not available, you may want to contact one of the cancer support organisations (see p.259).

## Coping with a visit to the breast clinic

- Make a list of questions and concerns you have. It is easy to forget things when you are feeling anxious.
- Consider taking along a relative or friend if you can to support you and to help you remember what was said – again it's easy to forget precise details, especially if you've had upsetting news.
- Dress in easy-to-remove separates, such as a shirt or jumper and pair of trousers or skirt, as you will have to strip off to your waist for some of the tests.
- Do not use talcum powder on the skin of your upper body as this can interfere with some tests such as an ultrasound scan or mammogram.
- Take a magazine or book to read. You may have to wait for long periods between different parts of the appointment.

## What are all the different tests and what do they involve?

### MAMMOGRAM

**What it is**

An X-ray of the breast. It involves taking two X-rays of each breast – one view of each breast on a vertical plane and one on a horizontal plane so as to view as much of the breast tissue as possible.

**When it is used**

To detect changes in the breast tissue, either as a routine screening procedure or when you or a doctor have detected visible or palpable changes such as a lump or thickening. If you are under 35, you will not usually be offered a mammogram unless you have signs or symptoms that could indicate breast cancer as your breasts will tend to be denser, making it more difficult to see changes.

**How it is done**

**Step 1** You will be asked to undress from the waist upwards.

**Step 2** The radiographer (the technician who takes the X-ray) will position you on the mammography machine with your arms carefully placed so they do not obstruct the X-ray. Each breast will be compressed between two X-ray plates first one way and then the other. It is necessary to get a picture of the whole breast tissue, including the 'tail' that extends into the armpit.

**Step 3** The radiographer will go behind a screen to shield themselves from the X-rays and take the mammograms.

**Step 4** You will be able to dress. You will usually be asked to wait a few minutes until the radiographer has examined the films to check that there are no technical problems.

The mammograms will be examined by a radiologist (a doctor who specialises in the use of X-ray and other forms of 'imaging' or scans for diagnosis and treatment) and a specialist cancer surgeon or physician in order to reach a diagnosis.

### Does it hurt?

Some women find having a mammogram quite uncomfortable, even painful, especially if they have particularly small or large breasts or if they have a tendency to tender breasts. Although mammography is not particularly pleasant, it only lasts a few seconds and cannot harm your breasts.

### BREAST ULTRASOUND SCAN

### What it is

A scan of the breast that uses high-frequency sound waves to detect changes in the breast tissue.

### When it is used

To detect the nature of the lump or thickening – whether it is solid or cystic (contains fluid) and, if solid, what the cause of the lump is. Ultrasound is better at picking up changes in the denser breast tissue of younger women, so you'll usually have an ultrasound scan rather than a mammogram if you are under 35.

### How it is done

The procedure is exactly the same as the scans used in pregnancy, except that having applied the ultrasound gel, the transducer is passed over your breasts rather than your abdomen. A scan is painless and takes just a few minutes.

**Step 1** You will be asked to undress to your waist.

**Step 2** You will lie down on an examination couch. The scan operator will spread a special gel that helps to conduct sound waves over your breasts (this may feel rather cold).

**Step 3** The scan operator will pass a small device (called a transducer) which emits sound waves over your breasts.

**Step 4** The echoes from your breast tissues are converted by a computer into an image of your breast tissue, which can be viewed on a monitor.

## DOPPLER ULTRASOUND

### What it is

A specialised type of ultrasound scan in which blood flow is shown up as areas of red or blue colour on a monitor.

### When it is done

To help the doctor decide if a lump is cancerous or benign, as one characteristic of cancerous lumps is that they have an increased blood supply.

### How it is done

As for ordinary ultrasound.

## FINE NEEDLE ASPIRATION

### What it is

The doctor draws off a sample of breast cells using a fine needle similar to the kind used to take a blood sample. The cells are sent to the laboratory to check for any signs of cancer.

### When it is used

To check if a lump or thickening is cancerous. It may also be used to drain fluid from a benign cyst.

### How it is done

The doctor inserts the needle into the lump or suspect area and draws off a sample of cells. This can be very uncomfortable momentarily. However, it takes less than a minute. It then takes about 15 minutes to an hour to prepare the cells for microscopic examination and to make a decision about whether or not they are cancerous.

## CORE BIOPSY

### What it is

This is a procedure in which a 'core' of suspicious tissue is removed for analysis. The needle is bigger than the one used for fine needle aspiration and you will be given a local anaesthetic.

**When it is used**

Core biopsy usually allows for a more accurate assessment than fine needle aspiration because the sample removed includes tissue from the lump and surrounding tissue, allowing the pathologist to compare the two. Some centres use core biopsy more frequently than others; different specialists have different views, so if you have any questions about why this procedure is being used in your case you should discuss them with your doctor. In most cases it will be done if:

- It is not clear from a fine needle aspiration whether the cells are cancerous.
- Fine needle aspiration has suggested benign disease but the doctor is still concerned it may be cancer.
- Fine needle aspiration has revealed cancer cells. A core biopsy enables the doctors to learn more about the nature of the tumour.

**How it is done**

Your skin and breast will be numbed with a local anaesthetic close to the lump or suspect area. When the anaesthetic has taken effect, a small cut is made in the skin of the breast. The doctor will then insert the needle through the cut and withdraw a section of tissue measuring approximately 10mm by 1 to 2mm. This isn't painful, but you may experience a sensation of pressure. At least four, sometimes more, core biopsies are usually taken through one incision.

In some units it is possible to get your results within 24 hours; however, it usually takes three days or more.

## EXCISION BIOPSY

**What it is**

The whole lump is removed under local or general anaesthetic.

**When it is used**

- Fine needle aspiration or core biopsy have not given a definite diagnosis.
- The surgeon is suspicious of the lump, even though the tests have suggested it is benign.
- You wish to have the lump removed.

**How it is done**

You may need to stay in hospital overnight, but in many hospitals excision biopsy is undertaken as a day case. It is usually done under a general anaesthetic, although some surgeons do offer local anaesthetic.

## Will the procedures be the same wherever I live and whichever hospital I go to?

Under the Government's National Cancer Plan, breast cancer care in England is organised in 34 local Cancer Networks, each of which has a catchment area of around 1.2 million people. Each Network has one or two key centres providing a full range of cancer diagnostic facilities and treatments, together with a number of other hospitals which provide more straightforward diagnostic facilities and treatments. Similar systems exist in Scotland and Wales. The idea is that no matter where you live you will be able to get the same diagnostic and treatment facilities without having to travel outside your area, although you may be referred to more than one hospital during the course of your treatment

## What other tests might be needed and why?

The tests performed at the clinic will usually give the doctor a preliminary answer as to whether or not you have cancer. However, sometimes further tests will be needed to reach a definite diagnosis. You may be offered Stereotactic biopsy and MRI mammography.

## STEREOTACTIC OR ULTRASOUND GUIDED BIOPSY

**What it is**

A way of getting a tissue or cell sample by fine needle aspiration or core biopsy, using mammography to view the breast and to guide the needle to the exact area from which cells or tissue are to be taken.

**When it is done**

When an abnormality that the doctor is unable to feel has been detected on the mammogram or ultrasound.

**What it involves**

**Step 1** You will be positioned on a mammography machine with a special device attached, all of which is linked to a computer. In most units you will be sitting down for this, although some units have special tables on which you will lie on your front.

**Step 2** In stereotactic biopsy, the radiographer will get a picture on a computer screen of the area from which the sample is to be taken.

**Step 3** The needle is guided by computer control so that its tip goes into the suspicious area that has been detected on the original mammogram.

The procedure can also be done using ultrasound guidance if the abnormal area can be seen on ultrasound.

The cell sample or tissue is then sent to the laboratory for analysis. Where the tissue sample has not been adequate to confirm or refute a diagnosis, you may occasionally need either a repeat core biopsy or a surgical biopsy. You may be recommended to have a follow-up mammogram six months after a stereotactic or ultrasound guided biopsy to ensure that no changes have occurred in the breast cells.

## MAGNETIC RESONANCE IMAGING
### What it is
MRI is a technique that produces high-quality cross-sectional or 3-D images using magnetism rather than X-ray or other radiation.
### When it is done
It may be recommended for you if:

- You are under 45 with an increased risk of developing breast cancer.
- You have had neoadjuvant therapy (see p.90) – i.e. you have been treated with chemotherapy to shrink a tumour before surgery. MRI will help your doctors decide how much tumour is left in the breast.
- The doctor is concerned you may have cancer, although other tests have failed to pick it up. In this case an MRI may be done before removing the lump to try to get further information.
- It is suspected cancer has recurred in your breast following a lumpectomy.
- You have had implants and there is a lump in your breast.
- You have a breast implant that, it is suspected, has leaked.

### If I am discovered to have breast cancer, what should a diagnosis include?
If you have had a core biopsy, the doctor should be able to tell you the type of cancer you have, the size of your tumour and where it is situated. Otherwise, once the lump or breast and lymph nodes have been removed, the doctor will also be able to tell you the type of cancer and whether there are any cancer cells present in the lymph nodes under your arm.

The tests you have had will also help your doctor to see the extent, or stage, of the cancer. The stage of a cancer describes its size and spread. The stage is combined with a grade. The grade is based on the appearance of the cells under a microscope and gives you an idea of how quickly the cancer is likely to develop. In one of the more common staging systems, there are four stages and three grades, explained below.

**Staging**

**Stage 1 tumours:** The tumour is less than two centimetres in diameter. This is usually a small, localised cancer: lymph glands in the armpit are not affected and there are no signs that the cancer has spread anywhere else.

**Stage 2 tumours:** This either means that the tumour measures between two and five centimetres, or the lymph glands in the armpit are affected, or both but there is no sign of the cancer spreading further.

**Stage 3 tumours:** The tumour is larger than five centimetres and may be attached to muscle, skin or other surrounding structures. In this stage of tumour the lymph glands are usually affected, but there are no signs that the cancer has spread beyond the breast or the lymph glands in the armpit.

**Stage 4 tumours:** This type of tumour may be of any size, but the lymph glands are usually affected and the cancer has spread to other parts of the body. This is secondary breast cancer.

**Grading**

**Grade 1:** low grade.

**Grade 2:** moderate grade.

**Grade 3:** high grade.

A low-grade tumour has cells that are very like normal breast cells. It is slow-growing and less likely to spread than a high-grade tumour. In high-grade tumours the cells are very abnormal and grow and spread quickly.

**Will diagnosis always be definite?**

In most cases it will be possible to tell you whether or not you have cancer. However, occasionally a definite diagnosis is not possible until the lump has been removed and analysed under a microscope.

**I've been told I have cancer 'in situ'. What does this mean?**

'In situ' disease is when the cells look like cancer cells but do not behave like cancer cells. They do not invade and spread into the surrounding tissues or beyond the breast. However, it is possible that invasive cancer may develop in these 'in situ' areas. 'In situ' cancer is confined to the milk channels or ducts in the breast. It is more commonly diagnosed in women following a routine mammogram because it is not usually big enough to be seen or felt. There are two types:

### DUCTAL CARCINOMA IN SITU (DCIS)

This is when these abnormal 'in situ' cells are present but contained within the breast or milk ducts. This is sometimes also referred to as intraductal cancer.

### LOBULAR CARCINOMA IN SITU (LCIS)

This is when changed cells are found within the lining of the lobules, the part of the breast where milk is manufactured and stored. It is possible for changed cells to be present in both breasts. LCIS is less common than DCIS and is not considered to be a breast cancer, but represents a risk factor. If you have LCIS but do not have any treatment, there is up to a 15 to 20 per cent risk that you will develop invasive breast cancer somewhere in either breast during the next 25 years. This type of in situ disease is very rarely found at a screening as it does not show on mammography.

### MICROCALCIFICATIONS

These are small deposits of calcium, either formed by rapidly dividing cells or by dying cells, that cannot be felt but that may be seen on a mammogram. When microcalcifications are concentrated in one area of the breast, it can be an early sign of breast cancer in situ or benign fibrocystic disease. Around 50 per cent of breast cancers detected by mammography appear as clusters of microcalcifications, while the remainder appear as masses or variations of normal breast tissue.

**The doctor said I had pre-cancerous changes. Does this mean I don't really have cancer?**

Sometimes doctors refer to in situ cancers as 'pre-invasive' or 'pre-cancerous'. Many experts think this is misleading. It is important to realise that in situ cancers are all 'non-invasive' at the time of diagnosis but many (although not all) in situ cancers have a risk of becoming invasive if left untreated.

**What are the different kinds of invasive breast cancer?**

## INVASIVE DUCTAL CANCER

It was originally thought that these cancers, which are the most common type (making up 70–80 per cent of all breast cancers diagnosed), arose from the breast ducts at the milk channels, which take the milk from the lobules where it is formed to the nipple. It is now known that most breast cancers – including invasive ductal cancers – arise in the lobule at the last branch of the ductal tree draining the duct, together known as the terminal duct lobular unit. Invasive ductal cancers are usually noticed as a lump and are either ordinary or of no special type cancers, or can have a particular pattern or are considered of a special type. Some special-type tumours such as tubular cancer (an uncommon type of ductal breast cancer named 'tubular' because of the way the cells look under the microscope) or mucinous cancer (a form of ductal carcinoma containing mucus-producing cells) have a better prognosis or outlook.

## INVASIVE LOBULAR CANCER

This arises in the lobule, and the cells are different in appearance to those of invasive ductal cancer. They can be more difficult to detect and are often noticeable as a thickening rather than a definite lump.

## INFLAMMATORY BREAST CANCER

Around 1 to 2 per cent of people with breast cancer develop a rare but fast-growing type of breast cancer known as inflammatory breast cancer. In this type of breast cancer the skin of the breast feels hot and looks red and inflamed, similar to a breast infection such as mastitis. The skin may also be ridged or pitted like the skin of an orange. This is known by the French term, *peau d'orange*. Other symptoms can include a lump or general swelling of the whole breast, pain in the breast or nipple, nipple discharge or inversion (turning in). The *peau d'orange* is caused by cancer cells blocking the channels through which lymph flows in the breast.

## PAGET'S DISEASE

This is another rare type of breast cancer, affecting fewer than 5 per cent of women with breast cancer. Men may also develop it, although this is extremely rare. Cancer cells travel from the ducts lying beneath the nipple onto the nipple itself, causing a red scaly rash which may spread to the areola (the dark area surrounding the nipple). In about half of all cases there is also a lump beneath the nipple. The rash may itch or burn and the nipple is sometimes inverted (pulled in) and there is usually a discharge. The symptoms can be confused with eczema or psoriasis. However, whereas Paget's Disease normally affects the nipple first, eczema usually affects the areola. Furthermore, Paget's Disease normally affects just one breast.

### What will happen next?

If you don't have cancer and don't need any further treatment, you will be able to go home. If cancer has been detected, one or more members of the breast care team will tell you in privacy what has been found. They should also give you some idea of the course of treatment likely to be recommended, although often you will be given a further appointment for this. If you are advised that you need an operation, you will either be given the date there and then or be sent the date by post.

### What if I'm told I have breast cancer?

However much you have prepared yourself it is usually a shock to be told you have breast cancer, and you are likely to need time for the news to sink in. You should have the opportunity to spend time with the breast care nurse, who can support you and help with any questions you may have (see p.47) and to discuss your cancer with family and friends, so that by the time any treatment begins you feel happy that it is the best option for you.

Some women deal with a diagnosis of breast cancer most effectively if they are fully informed about their cancer, and want to be involved in decision-making every step of the way. Others are happy to leave everything in the hands of the medical team. In between are those who want to be kept informed about the various procedures but are content to leave major decision-making to the doctors. You won't necessarily know which category you fall into until it happens. Shock can have a strange effect and even women who normally like to be well informed can find that when the time comes they prefer to leave it to the medical staff. However much you choose to be involved, no operation or procedure will be carried out without your informed written consent.

**If I'm diagnosed with breast cancer, does that mean my daughter(s) will get it too?**
Breast cancer is quite common, so just because you have been diagnosed with it doesn't mean your daughter(s) are at a higher risk. Some cancers do have an inherited component, however, and your diagnosis may increase your daughter's risk, although it is by no means certain she will develop cancer in the future. In order to assess your daughter's risk you need to consider:

- **Your age.** Breast cancer risk increases with age, so the older you are when you develop it, the lower your daughter's risk.
- **Whether the cancer affected one or both breasts.** An inherited risk is more likely if both breasts are affected.
- **Whether any of your close relatives have had breast cancer.** The risk increases with the number of relatives affected.
- **The age of your daughter.**
- **Whether your daughter has any risk factors of her own** (see p.8).

If you are worried, discuss these issues with your doctor, who can explain in more detail and, where necessary, refer your daughter(s) to a family breast clinic.

**I've heard that it's better to be treated in a hospital that has a multi-disciplinary breast cancer team and a specialised breast unit. Is this true?**
Research has shown that women treated in a specialised unit with a multi-disciplinary team – that is, a group of different specialists who meet regularly to discuss each person's case and share their expertise – do better both physically and psychologically. The Government

has incorporated this principle into its National Cancer Plan and all breast units should now have, or be working towards having, a multi-disciplinary breast team. A typical team will include:

- A breast surgeon (surgical oncologist), who is experienced in lumpectomy (wide local excision) and mastectomy and sometimes breast reconstruction.
- A medical oncologist (specialist in the drug treatment of cancer), who will plan chemotherapy, hormone therapy and other drug treatments.
- A radiotherapist (sometimes called a clinical oncologist), who is an expert in giving and planning any radiotherapy.
- A breast cancer nurse, who will support you throughout your breast cancer journey.
- Palliative care specialists: doctors and nurses who are experienced in the relief of unpleasant symptoms and side-effects and who help provide psychological support for people with all stages of cancer, including advanced breast cancer.

### Can I get a second opinion?

If you are in a hospital with a multi-disciplinary breast cancer team, all treatment will have been carefully planned by a group of different specialists. This is an ideal situation that unfortunately is still not available in every hospital. If you do not have access to a multi-disciplinary team or you are not happy with your doctor or do not feel happy with the proposed course of treatment, you have the right to ask for a second opinion. Of course, you will want to know what your surgeon's speciality is – they should be either a general surgeon with a declared breast sub-speciality interest or a surgeon who specialises entirely in breast surgery. If this is not the case, then you should ask for a referral to a breast specialist. Bear in mind that it can take time to set up an appointment with another doctor, so it is important to be sure exactly why you want another opinion and what you expect to gain from such a consultation. If you do decide to opt for a second opinion, it's a good idea to take a friend or relative with you. It is also a good idea to take a list of questions with you so that you can ensure all your concerns have been covered.

## Questions to ask your doctor

- What kind of breast cancer do I have?
- How common is my kind of breast cancer?
- How big is the tumour?
- How will I know whether or not the disease has begun to spread?
- Will I need any further tests before a treatment plan is decided?
- If I am on the Pill or HRT, should I carry on taking it?
- If I have to stop taking the Pill, what alternatives do I have?
- Does the fact I have breast cancer increase the risk for any other members of my family, ie my mother, sister or daughter?
- Is there anything I can do to improve my health, i.e. stopping smoking or eating a healthier diet, before I start treatment?

## I want to get things over with as quickly as possible. Can I speed things up?

Once you have been diagnosed, it's natural to want to get treatment over and done with as quickly as possible so you can get on with your life. Unfortunately, although there have been improvements in the availability of staff and equipment, there is a lot of pressure on breast cancer services, and in some areas of the UK it may be impossible to avoid a wait. Your doctor will take into account the type of cancer you have, how it is likely to progress and your individual situation to prevent you having to wait too long for essential treatment. If you are worried about waiting, you should discuss how long you are likely to have to wait and how this might affect your chances of remaining cancer free in the long term with your doctor or breast cancer nurse. Short delays of a few weeks will not affect your outcome, although some studies have shown that delays of three months or more may be associated with a less favourable outcome, so treatment should definitely begin within this time frame.

## I feel like it's all going too fast. Can I slow things down?

If there are no particular reasons for urgent treatment, it should be possible to delay things for a few weeks without any harmful effects if you feel things are going too fast, giving you time to discuss your options, have further consultations and come to terms with the proposed treatments. However, if you have a type of cancer that tends to spread quickly, such as Inflammatory Breast Cancer, the doctor will usually recommend starting treatment promptly. You may feel overwhelmed and that it is all out of your control. You should feel free to ask the doctor or breast nurse about anything you are worried about. It may also help to talk to other women who have had the same kind of cancer or to a counsellor. The breast care nurse may be able to arrange this or suggest how you might arrange it yourself.

### I don't like my consultant. Can I ask to see a different one?

It is important for you to have confidence in the person in charge of your treatment. However, in some instances there may be a personality clash or some other reason why you do not feel happy with him or her. In this case you have the right to a second opinion and the option of having your care transferred to another consultant. There are three ways to go about this:

**1.** Tell the consultant that you would like a second opinion or to be transferred. If you feel able, try to explain why, as this may be of help to the consultant and any future patients.

**2.** If you don't feel able to tell your consultant face to face, speak to your GP, explain what the problem is and what you would like done.

**3.** If you have a breast care nurse, discuss it with her. She should be able to liaise with your consultant and/or GP as necessary.

### What if I feel my condition is getting worse while I wait for treatment?

If you feel that the lump is getting bigger, then let the doctor who is treating you know.

### Will I get better treatment if I go privately?

The 'hotel' side of private care – the hospital environment, your room, meals and other services – will almost certainly be superior to that of the NHS. The surgeon may also have more time to spend with you. However, if you are seen in an NHS hospital with a multi-disciplinary breast team, the treatment you receive should be at least as good if not better than in a private hospital. Many private hospitals have no medical staff on duty at night, so you may well be better off in an NHS hospital where there is back-up should you need it. The most important thing is to be treated by a specialised breast team.

# Starting treatment

Different treatments and when they are offered will depend on the type of breast cancer you have, where it is situated, its size and whether it has invaded surrounding breast tissue with the potential to spread to other parts of your body. Breast cancer treatments can be divided into two main kinds:

**Local treatments**

This is treatment aimed at the breast itself and the axillary lymph nodes. Its aim is to try to eradicate the cancer from the breast and lymph nodes before it spreads. Local therapies include surgery such as lumpectomy, mastectomy and lymph node removal and treatments such as radiotherapy.

**Adjuvant treatments**

These are designed to eradicate any cancer cells that may have spread (metastasised) from the breast to other parts of the body. These treatments therefore increase your chances of remaining cancer free in the long term and include chemotherapy and hormonal therapies.

Local and adjuvant therapies are usually combined to ensure that your cancer is treated as comprehensively as possible.

## Will the different treatments be explained?

You will usually have a meeting with one or more members of the breast care team (typically a surgeon and a breast care nurse) at diagnosis or shortly afterwards. At this consultation the various different treatment options should be discussed and explained, together with their pros and cons.

### Questions to ask your doctor

- What treatments are you proposing to treat my cancer with?
- Why do you consider these treatments appropriate?
- What are the advantages of this treatment for me personally?
- Are there any alternatives?
- What are the aims of treatment?
- What are the benefits of treatment?
- What side-effects might I expect?

- What are the long-term implications of treatment, for example, early menopause?
- How long am I likely to need to stay in hospital?
- Will I be offered adjuvant treatment?

## How will the breast care team decide which treatments to offer me?

The team will try to decide which treatment plan has the best chance of eradicating or controlling your cancer. In deciding the most appropriate course of treatment for you, the doctors have to consider factors to do with the cancer and factors to do with you and the likely interaction between them. Factors taken into account will include:

- The size of the tumour and how much it has progressed.
- The grade of the tumour.
- What your cancer cells look like under a microscope (their histological appearance: the grade and pattern); how different they are to normal breast cells and whether they look as if they are slow- or fast-growing; whether or not the tumour is seen to penetrate blood or lymphatic vessels.
- Whether it has spread to the axillary lymph nodes (see p.54).
- Whether the cells have receptors for certain hormones or other proteins on the cell surface (see p.95).
- Your age.
- Whether you have been through the menopause.
- Your overall health.

## How much choice am I likely to have about treatment?

In some cases the most appropriate course of treatment will be clear-cut. However, in others it may not be. In hospitals where there is a multi-disciplinary team (see p.41) your case will have been discussed and the expertise of all the various medical experts brought to bear on treatment options. You should have the opportunity to be involved in your treatment planning as much or as little as you like. If you don't feel happy with the treatment proposed, you may wish to explore other options and may wish to consider getting a second opinion.

## What should I expect from the treatments offered?

All treatments have risks as well as benefits. You will need to establish what the proposed treatment is expected to achieve in your particular case in order to decide whether or not it is best for you.

### Questions to ask your doctor

- How long has this particular treatment been used?
- What outcome can I expect?
- How invasive is the treatment?
- What side-effects can I expect?
- How disruptive is it likely to be to my lifestyle?

## Will I have access to a breast care nurse?

You are likely to see a whole range of different medical staff throughout your cancer treatment. Through it all, in an NHS hospital, the breast care nurse is often the one person who remains the same. She will become familiar with your case and will be present at meetings of the breast team when your treatment or progress is discussed. If you are being treated in a major cancer centre at one of the larger hospitals, there will almost certainly be one or more breast care nurses on the spot whom you can turn to for advice, information, counselling and help with any of your concerns at any time during and after treatment. If you are being treated in a smaller hospital within your local network, the breast care nurse(s) might travel to the hospital from the major hospital in your area. You may be assigned to a particular nurse, although you can of course consult any of the team.

## How the breast care nurse can help you

She will see you at diagnosis and in hospital before, during and after treatment to make sure you understand your diagnosis and treatment and to answer any questions you may have. She may also see you when you come in for other treatments.

- She can help you decide between reconstruction and wearing an external prosthesis and may have before and after photos of other patients and a few sample prostheses for you to look at.
- She will usually be there at your first follow-up clinic after surgery to go through the results with you. She may also be present at subsequent follow-ups.

- She may have a special interest in complementary therapies and be able to refer you to a suitable therapist or support group.
- She can talk to your partner or your children if they need help or advice.
- Breast care nurses carry a bleeper or pager so you can consult her if you have any queries. In some units you may be given a dedicated number you can call to speak to a nurse or leave a message on an answer-phone.
- Some breast care nurse teams keep a library from which you can obtain leaflets or borrow books, tapes, videos and other sources of information.
- Some breast care nurses organise support groups for women once they leave the hospital and may be able to organise for you to speak to someone who has had the same kind of cancer or treatments. If there aren't breast care nurses at your hospital, you may want to contact one of the support or patient groups listed on pages 259–60.

**What are the surgical options?**

Most women with breast cancer will need some kind of surgery initially. The basic choice is between a lumpectomy (wide local excision), where just the lump or area of abnormal cells is removed together with some surrounding normal tissue to achieve clear margins, and a mastectomy, where the whole breast is removed.

### LUMPECTOMY (wide local excision)

Provided your cancer has been detected at an early stage and is suitable in other ways, the surgeon will usually try to conserve your breast by performing a lumpectomy (wide local excision). At the same operation you will also have axillary lymph node sampling/dissection (see p.54) or removal of most of your axillary nodes to check whether your cancer has spread. Subsequently, radiotherapy is given as an essential part of breast-conserving treatment and is designed to kill any stray cancer cells. Without radiotherapy there is a strong risk that the cancer could recur in the affected breast, even when the cancer has been completely removed.

## MASTECTOMY

This is an operation to remove all of the breast tissue. Various types may be performed depending on what kind of tumour you have, how large it is, where in the breast it is situated and whether it has invaded surrounding tissue. The options are:

- **Total or simple mastectomy:** All the breast tissue is removed but not the lymph glands.

- **Modified radical mastectomy (also called Patey mastectomy):** Removal of all of the breast plus all axillary lymph nodes under the arm (this is known as axillary clearance). The pectoral muscles are not usually removed.

- **Radical mastectomy:** The breast and axillary lymph nodes are removed together with the chest wall muscles. This operation is not often required and is very rarely performed nowadays.

- **Subcutaneous mastectomy:** The breast tissue is removed except for the nipple and areola and the bulk is replaced with a prosthesis. This carries more risk as it leaves areas that may still be affected, but may be used for some women with a strong family history asking for a prophylactic mastectomy.

### Questions to ask your doctor

- What are my options for surgery?
- Is breast-conserving surgery (lumpectomy) an option?
- Which type of surgery do you recommend?
- What are the risks of surgery?
- What are your results in terms of complications and recurrence?
- Will my lymph nodes be removed? Which operation will you perform?
- How am I likely to feel after the operation?
- What will I have to do to care for my wound after I get home?
- Where will the scar(s) be? What will they look like?
- Are there any options on where the scar will be?
- Will I be able to keep my nipple?
- If I keep my nipple, will its position be affected?
- Is there anything I can do beforehand to prepare my skin?
- How soon can I get back to my normal activities?
- Which specialists should I see before deciding on treatment?
- Is there anyone I can talk to who has had the same surgery as me?

# A breast care nurse's perspective

My remit is to all women who have, or think they have, breast cancer. This means I have contact with many women who ultimately will have benign disease. Their anxieties are as great as those that end up with breast cancer, and they need to air these feelings.

Psychological care for those with breast cancer is the biggest aspect of our role. We know that some women with breast cancer have high levels of anxiety, depression and sexual dysfunction following their diagnosis, and these problems will only increase if left untreated, so it is vital that we meet these women regularly to assess them for these disorders. We are able to refer them to an appropriate therapist, counsellor or their GP.

All women have some levels of anxiety at the time of their cancer diagnosis and though their treatments. An important way of reducing this anxiety and distress is to give information about their disease and the possible treatments that they will need.

This information has to be given sensitively, and as the patient requires it. Some need to know everything, including statistics about outcomes; others only require the basic information about their treatments as they go along.

In our centre, I am present in the One-Stop Clinics when the women come in with their breast problems. I try to meet them all, even before their diagnosis, so that I have begun to establish their trust and confidence. In this clinic, they receive provisional results of a fine needle aspiration (FNA), mammogram and ultrasound scan. A benign patient is reassured and discharged from the clinic. A breast cancer patient is warned that she probably has got the disease, but that we need confirmation of this from the FNA. She is given any information that she requires at the time and our contact number so that she can ring us if she wishes.

I am present when she and her family come back to the clinic. The consultant will confirm the diagnosis and discuss the treatments with her and her family in more detail. A date will be arranged for the surgery. I can then take her into a quiet room where we can go over the information she has been given and I can provide literature about the treatments, put her in touch with volunteers if she wishes and allow her to air her fears. Between this clinic and her admission, I will normally make contact with her again, either with a phone call, a meeting in my office or a home visit.

I visit the woman on the ward pre-operatively to go through wound management and what she can expect to do when she gets home. Two weeks after her surgery, we meet again with the consultant, who will give her the results of her surgery and the decision that has been made about her adjuvant treatments.

For some, treatments are not 'black and white' and time needs to be given to discuss the options so that the patient can make informed decisions. Decisions have to be made about chemotherapy, entering clinical trials, whether she wants a breast reconstruction and whether or not she wants conventional medicine at all. My role is vital in providing the time needed for the woman to make these decisions.

Throughout any or all of these treatments I stay in touch with the woman. She knows she can contact me at any time if she has any queries or concerns and that her access to me is not limited to her treatment time only but at any time in the future. I am able to refer the woman back to the appropriate help for whatever concerns she has, and I can also direct her towards our support groups and alternative therapies.

As a breast care nurse I liase with the Multi-Disciplinary Team on behalf of my patients so that their journey is, hopefully, smooth and as stress-free as possible.

## How long will I have to stay in hospital if I have surgery?

A lot will depend on the type of surgery, whether you experience any complications and your overall state of health. Lumpectomy can be done on a day surgery basis, although you or your surgeon may prefer you to stay in hospital overnight. If an axillary node operation is also performed, the hospital stay may range from two to five days. After mastectomy or axillary clearance, the average stay is five to seven days. However, some people go home on the first day with a couple of drains left in place and with arrangements for a district nurse to visit each day to empty them.

## How has the doctor decided whether to offer me lumpectomy (wide local excision) or mastectomy?

**Lumpectomy:** You will usually be offered a lumpectomy (or wide local excision, to use the correct medical term) if:

- Your tumour is less than 4 cm in diameter, although this will also depend on the size of the tumour in relation to the size of your breast.
- You have a single small tumour.
- You have a localised area of ductal carcinoma in situ (DCIS).

The question of how large an area of normal breast cells surrounding tissue needs to be clear of disease is a subject of great debate among doctors. However, many experts aim to clear an area of 1 cm around the abnormal tissue.

**Mastectomy:** The doctor may recommend you have a mastectomy if:

- The tumour is more than 4 cm in diameter.
- More than one cancer has been detected in your breast.
- You have extensive ductal carcinoma in situ. Again, just how extensive is a matter of debate; some doctors will recommend this if the affected area is 4 cm or more, others if it is 2.5 cm or more, depending on the site(s) and size of the breast.
- The cancer affects the nipple or the area beneath it. However, again, this is controversial. Many surgeons will still offer breast conservation surgery, removing the nipple and areola (area around the nipple) with or without some reconstruction to get the best possible appearance.

## Will I be given any choice in the type of surgery recommended?

Often you will be given a choice of breast-conserving surgery or mastectomy, with or without breast reconstruction (see p.69). Information on options is available from your doctor, breast care nurse, relatives and friends, or seek more information from books, cancer organisations or the Internet. There is no single correct choice for everyone; it is a question of coming to a decision that you feel most comfortable with. The one you decide upon will depend on many different factors, such as how prepared you feel to deal with the effects and side-effects of different kinds of surgery, as well as individual factors such as your age, your personality, your relationships and how you feel about your body.

### Questions you might want to consider

- How do you feel about your breasts? How important are they to your self-esteem?
- Are you likely to feel less feminine without a breast?
- How disruptive is treatment likely to be to your everyday life? How long is it likely to take? If you work, how much time will you need to take off? How much time are you able to take off ?
- What are the likely side-effects and how likely are they to make it difficult to carry on with your life?
- What kind of follow-up will be necessary?

### Mastectomy vs Lumpectomy

Mastectomy

Pros

- You may be able to avoid radiotherapy (see pages 63–64 for benefits and risks).
- You may feel you are 'getting the cancer out of your system'. If this feeling is persistent, you may want to choose mastectomy. But bear in mind that fear of recurrence is a reality for most women following breast cancer, whatever kind of surgery they have had.
- Whether immediate or delayed, breast reconstruction can produce extremely good cosmetic results, although the reconstructed breast will not have normal sensation (see p.73).

## Cons

- Feelings of loss.
- Potential change in the way you view yourself and your body.
- Potential loss of confidence that may affect other aspects of your life and relationships.

### Lumpectomy

### Pros

- A more acceptable cosmetic result because your breast is preserved.
- There is likely to be less change in the way you view your body, resulting in higher self-esteem and confidence.
- No need to buy special clothes.

### Cons

- The need for three to six weeks of radiotherapy, necessitating daily hospital appointments.
- The potential side-effects of radiotherapy (see pages 63–4).
- Your skin may change in texture because of radiotherapy.
- The risk and anxiety of a possible local recurrence in your breast.
- You may need a further operation if the margins of the excision are found to contain cancerous cells.

### Does the timing of surgery affect my chances of staying cancer free?

It has been suggested that for pre-menopausal women the point in the menstrual cycle at which surgery is performed may influence the likelihood of cancer recurring. However, the importance of this remains unclear and other studies suggest that timing is unimportant. If you are concerned, discuss the issue with your surgeon, who should be aware of the research results, although most units do not time surgery in relation to the menstrual cycle.

### I've been told I will need axillary node surgery. What is this?

The axillary nodes are lymph nodes (sometimes also called glands) under your armpit or axilla (see explanation below). Some or all of the axillary nodes will be removed at the same time as your breast surgery to check whether they contain any cancer cells. If some of the nodes are removed, this is known as axillary node sampling. If a more comprehensive dissection takes place, it is known as axillary node clearance.

## Why is it done?

The body's tissues are bathed in a watery fluid called lymph, derived from the bloodstream. Lymph, along with cells and other small particles such as bacteria, is transported in the lymphatic system, which is part of your body's immune system and helps defend you against infection and disease. At various points along the lymphatic system are nodes: filters that trap micro-organisms and other foreign bodies travelling in the lymph. The nodes contain lymphocytes, a type of white blood cell which destroys invading bacteria and viruses. Cancer cells too can spread via the lymphatic system if they break off the original tumour. The nearest lymph nodes to the breast are the 20 or so axillary nodes under your arm. There are also lymph nodes behind the breastbone, where the ribs join, and at the base of the neck above the collarbone. Removing the axillary lymph nodes and examining them under a microscope determines whether any cells have spread from the breast and the likelihood of distant spread into other parts of your body, which helps the breast care team to plan the most appropriate further treatment.

## Does everyone with breast cancer need lymph node removal?

The majority do, although if you have an in situ cancer the lymph nodes will not need to be removed.

## Are there other ways of detecting whether cancer has spread to the lymph nodes and which are affected?

A newer method of checking potential spread to the lymph nodes is currently being researched. Known as Sentinel Node Biopsy, it involves injecting a small amount of radioactive liquid around the cancerous area before surgery. A scan is then done of the nodes to see which have taken up the radioactive liquid. At surgery a blue dye is also injected around the cancer and is taken up into the draining lymph channels and moves to the sentinel node or nodes. Only nodes that are radioactive or blue, the so-called 'sentinel' nodes, are then removed and checked for cancerous cells. When fully evaluated, it is hoped that this will prove an effective way to tell whether any lymph nodes are affected. Treatment – either removing the remaining lymph nodes or giving radiotherapy – could then be restricted to patients with cancer in one of these sentinel nodes.

### Are there any alternatives to surgery?

Most doctors consider that surgery is the best way of eliminating breast cancer. In some instances you may be offered chemotherapy, hormonal therapy or sometimes radiotherapy before surgery (see pages 89 and 94). In a few cases, for example if you have other medical problems that might make surgery inadvisable or dangerous, chemotherapy or hormonal therapy may be used instead.

### Will I need any tests or other procedures before undergoing surgery?

Before undergoing surgery you may be given a chest X-ray, an analysis of your blood count and blood chemistry and an analysis of your urine to check on your general state of health, the function of your liver and kidneys and your body's ability to tolerate surgery and anaesthesia. If the lymph nodes are enlarged and your doctors think they may be involved, or if you have a large cancer or in cases where the skin is affected (ulceration or *peau d'orange*) or the cancer involves underlying ribs or muscles, you may be given a bone scan and a body scan to see whether there is any evidence of spread. However, this is not used for assessing the stage of most early breast cancers.

### Are there any risks or any complications from surgery?

Any kind of surgery carries a small risk of complications. General complications can include deep vein thrombosis and pulmonary embolism (blood clot formation in the legs or lungs), although you will be given injections and may also have to wear elastic stockings to combat this. Getting up and about as quickly as possible will help avoid this. Some specific complications of breast surgery are listed below. Although it may look daunting to see them grouped together like this, bear in mind that complications are unusual and you are unlikely to experience all of them. What's more, they can all be managed and treated very effectively.

#### Infection

This is a risk with any kind of wound, although it is unusual following breast cancer surgery. An infection can develop anything from a few days after surgery to around two to three weeks later when the wound has healed. It is more likely to occur if you have had a larger operation or reconstruction, and in this case 'prophylactic' antibiotics may be prescribed after the operation to prevent infection from occurring. Smokers and diabetics are more likely to suffer wound infections.

**Signs and symptoms include:**

- Increased soreness, redness or warmth around the wound or dressing.
- Increased tenderness or swelling.
- Leaking from the wound.
- A rise in your temperature, together with a general feeling of being unwell.

If you do notice any of these, report them to the doctor, who may prescribe a course of antibiotics to clear up the infection.

### Haematoma

This is the accumulation of blood within the tissues around the incision which can cause swelling, discomfort and hardness. Like a bruise, the skin will be discoloured. If the blood clots, it can form a hard lump under the skin. The body will eventually reabsorb the blood, although this can take some time and can cause scar tissue to form. If a haematoma is large, it may have to be removed in an operation, but sometimes it is possible to draw off the fluid using a syringe.

### Seroma

This is an accumulation of fluid in the tissues in the breast or beneath the arm, where lymph nodes have been removed or, if you have had a mastectomy, it may be fluid on the chest wall. The fluid, which is usually clear and straw-coloured, is slowly reabsorbed as new lymphatic channels form. Before this happens, fluid may collect under the wound and cause discomfort, but it can be drawn off easily and painlessly by syringe. Seromas can be left alone if they are not giving you any symptoms. Sometimes fluid leaks from the wound. In this case, put a padding over the top of your dressing and report it to the doctor.

### Cording

Raised cord, like strings of fibrous tissue, can develop down the arm or side of the body. Although not harmful, cording can be uncomfortable and restrict movement. It is thought to be a result of clotted or thrombosed lymph vessels. Cording usually develops from six to eight weeks after surgery, but can appear several months afterwards. Cords tend to disappear of their own accord, but this can take many months. A physiotherapist can show you exercises that can help stretch the cords and prevent restriction of movement.

## Scar tissue

As the wound heals, a scar will form. This may be felt as a hard lumpy area beneath the skin, although as healing proceeds it will tend to get more compact. The exact shape and size will depend on the nature of the lump and how much tissue has been removed. The feeling of scar tissue can alarm some women, who fear that the cancer may have returned. If you are worried, contact the breast nurse or surgeon who should be able to reassure you. As healing continues, the scar tissue may pull on surrounding skin causing it to pucker. To try to avoid this happening, keep your skin supple by massaging the area with an emollient cream or lotion.

## Lymphoedema

The removal of lymph nodes from under the arm slows the flow of lymphatic fluid. This fluid may accumulate in the arm and hand, causing uncomfortable swelling. Less often the fluid accumulates in the breast, chest area, the shoulder or the area behind the armpit. This may happen immediately after treatment but in some instances lymphoedema doesn't develop until many years later. Lymphoedema affects around a quarter to a third of those who have had surgery and/or radiotherapy for breast cancer, although why some women develop it and not others is still a mystery.

If your arm, hand, fingers or chest wall appear swollen, report it to the doctor or breast nurse, who should be able to reassure you that there is no more sinister reason for the swelling and treat you, or in some hospitals refer you to a nurse who specialises in the management of lymphoedema. The aim of treatment is to reduce swelling and to encourage the rest of your lymphatic system to work more efficiently. Symptoms can usually be controlled by a combination of self-help measures (see below) and by wearing an elastic sleeve to compress the arm and reduce the swelling. A massage technique known as manual lymphatic drainage can often encourage the lymphatic fluid to disperse. The sooner any swelling is treated the better and the nurse can teach you a simplified form of this massage to do at home.

## Is it possible to prevent lymphoedema?

Although it may not be possible to prevent lymphoedema completely, you may be able to reduce the risk of it occurring. Exercise and activity help the lymphatic system to work more effectively, so you should try to keep your arm moving following treatment. You should also protect the arm and hand on the treated side from injury and pressure which can encourage lymph to accumulate.

- Try to use your arm as normally as possible to encourage lymph to drain and prevent joint stiffness.
- Contact your GP immediately if you suspect any infection (see above).
- Avoid very hot water as this can increase swelling.
- Take care of your skin. Moisturise daily with a non-perfumed cream or lotion.
- Insect bites can exacerbate problems. In summer or on holiday, use an insect repellent cream or spray.
- Avoid sunburn by using a high SPF sunscreen.
- Cuts, scratches, bites or other injuries to the arm or hand can slightly increase the risk of lymphoedema developing so take precautions to avoid them. For example, wear gloves for washing up and/or gardening.
- If you do suffer a cut, scratch or bite, treat it promptly by washing it and applying an antiseptic.
- Avoid tight bra straps and anything that constricts your arm or hand, such as tight sleeves, tight rings or heavy bags.
- Avoid having injections e.g. vaccinations in the affected arm.
- If you need to have your blood pressure measured, ask for the cuff to be placed on your other arm.
- Be careful to avoid nicks and cuts when shaving under your arms. It is best to use an electric razor or depilatory cream.
- Be careful to avoid damage to cuticles when cutting your nails or having them manicured.

## I feel pressured into having a mastectomy. Can I have a lumpectomy (wide local excision) instead, and will this be safe?

Ideally your doctor and/or breast care nurse will explain all the various options so that you can be as involved in the decision as you want to be. The important thing to bear in mind is that lumpectomy (wide local excision) with radiotherapy is just as effective as mastectomy in most cases in achieving local control.

## How can I find out more information about the surgeon who is going to do my operation?

This can be difficult as there are no centrally held or local records. The website www.drfoster.co.uk has details of doctors. Essentially it will be up to you to ask questions. These could include:

- Are you a breast specialist or a general surgeon?
- Do you have any areas of special expertise and interest?
- Who is in your breast team and is it a multi-disciplinary team?
- How many people with breast cancer do you treat per year?
- Will I see a medical oncologist and a clinical oncologist before and/or after surgery has been carried out?
- How many operations of the type you are recommending do you carry out a year?
- What is your complication rate and what complications have occurred in previous patients?
- What is your local recurrence rate and how does this compare with other hospitals/national figures?

## What is radiotherapy?

Radiotherapy is a method of treating cancer using high-energy X-rays to destroy the cells. There are two main types – external and internal (see below).

## In what circumstances might the doctor recommend radiotherapy?

Radiotherapy is likely to be recommended if you have had a lumpectomy to reduce the risk of recurrence in the affected breast or if you have had a mastectomy and the doctor considers there is a risk of some residual cancer cells remaining that might lead to a recurrence. If lymph node clearance has been performed, you won't usually need radiotherapy to the armpit. However, if only a few nodes have been removed and were found to contain cancer cells or if no lymph nodes have been removed, radiotherapy or further surgery may be used to treat the nodes in your armpit.

## Questions to ask your doctor

- Why do I need radiotherapy?
- What are the risks and side-effects?
- What are the long-term effects?
- When will treatment start?
- How is radiotherapy likely to affect me?
- How can I look after myself during radiotherapy?
- How will my breast look after radiotherapy?
- How successful is radiotherapy likely to be in stopping the cancer from recurring in my breast?

## When is treatment likely to begin?

Ideally radiotherapy should begin about four to six weeks after surgery, unless you are having chemotherapy as well, which is usually given before radiotherapy. Treatments are usually given every day – or sometimes every other day – from Monday to Friday and this regime usually lasts for three to six weeks.

Currently some women are having to wait six to 12 weeks before treatment can start as a result of nationwide shortages of equipment and staff. It is not known whether these delays in treatment increase the chances of a cancer recurring, although the risk is thought to be fairly small. However, it is undoubtedly distressing to have to wait for treatment, especially when you want to get on with your life. If you are feeling upset, contact your breast cancer nurse or doctor to discuss your feelings and possible options.

## How is the treatment actually given?

### External radiotherapy

In this form of radiotherapy, high-energy X-ray beams are directed to the breast and/or armpits by a radiotherapy machine to kill off any stray cancer cells. Treatment is given in the hospital radiotherapy department, usually on an outpatient basis unless you are already an inpatient.

### Internal radiotherapy (brachytherapy)

In this form of radiotherapy, radioactive wires are inserted into the breast tissue under general anaesthetic. This allows an extra dose of radiotherapy to be delivered to the area surrounding the tumour. You will have to stay in hospital and be nursed in a separate room to limit radiation exposure to others. Nursing staff and visitors may be limited to prevent them coming into contact with radiation and you will not be allowed to be in contact with children and pregnant women. Once the wires have been removed, the radioactivity disappears.

### What can I expect when I go for treatment?

You can usually expect to make one or two preliminary visits lasting about half an hour to an hour to plan the treatment, followed by the actual treatment.

### What is treatment planning and why do I need it?

It is important that radiotherapy is given accurately to ensure all possible cancer cells are treated. The doctors will plan your course of treatment carefully, based on your individual needs.

**Step 1** You will be asked to undress from the waist upwards.

**Step 2** You will be asked to lie under a simulator with your hands holding a bar above your head. This is a machine that moves in exactly the same way as a radiotherapy machine but takes X-rays rather than giving treatment. This gives the radiotherapist or clinical oncologist a record of the exact area to be treated.

**Step 3** The radiographer will measure the area and draw lines around it with a felt-tip pen to show where the X-ray beams are to be aimed. You will have to lie extremely still while this is done. The marks will probably disappear before you start treatment.

**Step 4** The simulator will be rotated to check the marks are in the correct position. The lights will be dimmed and the simulator will then move around you taking X-rays. If the lymph nodes are also being treated, more X-rays will be done. The whole process can take 30 to 40 minutes. The radiographer will also take Polaroid pictures of the marks.

**Step 5** The films will be checked and the radiographer will make three to five tiny permanent pinprick marks (tattoos). These will be used to make sure you are always in the correct position on the treatment machine.

**Step 6** The radiographer will measure the contours of your chest wall using light beams projected against your skin, a process that lasts about five minutes.

## What can I expect at treatment visits?

Treatment will usually start a few days after planning and is much faster and simpler. The whole process usually takes only about 10 to 15 minutes.

**Step 1** The radiographer will position you carefully on the couch and put your arm into place as before so that the machine can deliver the rays effectively.

**Step 2** The radiographer will then leave the room and switch on the radiotherapy machine for about a minute.

## Is it painful?

Radiotherapy isn't painful, but some women find it uncomfortable to stay still and hold their arm in position, especially if lymph nodes have been removed. It can help to practise beforehand by lying on your bed with a pillow or two placed vertically beneath your neck and shoulders, then place your hands on your head and allow your elbows to relax at right angles. Sometimes the treatment can make your muscles and shoulder joint stiff. The breast care nurse or physiotherapist can show you some exercises to help ease stiffness.

## How is radiotherapy likely to affect me?

As with chemotherapy, radiotherapy affects normal cells as well as cancer cells. Fortunately, normal cells are better able to recover than cancer cells. However, they may become damaged either in the short or longer term. Everyone responds differently, but certain side-effects are common. These include sunburn-like symptoms such as reddening, itching, skin soreness, increased pigmentation and peeling and flaking. Other women notice twinges and sharp shooting pains in the area. If the area treated includes the middle part of your chest, you may experience heartburn. More rarely you may experience loss of appetite and nausea. Fatigue is also extremely common, especially as treatment continues. Although most of these symptoms disappear when treatment is stopped, fatigue can sometimes last for months afterwards. There is also a risk of depression, which in itself can make you feel fatigued. If you are experiencing these side-effects and don't feel able to cope, contact your breast nurse or one of the organisations listed on pages 259–60 for support.

## Coping with radiotherapy

- Wear loose clothing that will not rub the irradiated area.
- Try not to allow the treated area to become too dry. Apply an unperfumed moisturising cream (check with the nurse or radiographer if you want to use a particular cream or lotion).
- Avoid using perfumed soaps, talcum powder, deodorants, body lotion or perfume during the course of treatment as these can make the skin sore.
- Try not to rub the skin as this can also cause soreness. If itching becomes a problem, the doctor can prescribe a mild (1%) hydrocortisone cream.
- Try to get a friend or relative to drive you to appointments or take a taxi, as you are likely to feel tired.
- Try to cut down on appointments, work and social activities until the course of treatment is over and you are feeling less tired.
- Consult the doctor if you develop any after-effects such as arm or rib pain or breathlessness following treatment.

## Are there likely to be longer-term effects?

Twinges, aches and shooting pains in the arm or hand on the side treated are quite common in the months following surgery and radiotherapy. Your breast may also feel tender and be slightly swollen and pink, or it may harden slightly. These symptoms are a sign that your body is healing and usually disappear over time, although a few women experience problems indefinitely. More rarely you may experience breathlessness and a dry cough caused by inflammation of the lung. If you do develop this, let your doctor know as there are treatments for it, although it will usually go away in time.

## Are there any serious long-term side-effects?

Rarely, there may be some serious, permanent side-effects. These include nerve pain, tingling, weakness and sometimes loss of movement, caused by damage to the nerves in the arm. There may also be fibrosis (build-up of scar tissue) within the lung or lining of the lung, causing a dry cough or breathlessness. Occasionally, weakening of the bones can lead to fracture of the ribs or collarbone. Lower dosages of radiation and improvements in the way treatment is planned and delivered mean that such side-effects are much rarer today than in the past. However, if you are worried, discuss your concerns with the radiologist.

**Is it true that radiotherapy increases the risk of heart disease?**
In a small number of women – fewer than one in 100 – radiotherapy may very slightly increase the risk of heart disease. This will usually be if your breast cancer was in your left breast, in which case the area treated may lie very close to the heart. In many cases special shields can be used to protect the heart. However, it is not always possible to guard the tip of the heart, which is situated close to the divide of the front left chest wall. In this case the doctor will weigh up the benefits of therapy against the slightly increased risk of causing heart problems and will discuss this with you before going ahead.

**Can radiotherapy affect the appearance of my breast?**
If your breast has been preserved, radiotherapy can make the skin drier and thinner in the area where the tumour was. You may also notice small, red, thread-like marks caused by the small blood vessels called capillaries becoming dilated. With modern techniques this is usually uncommon and although unsightly it is not harmful. A few women (around three in 10) notice that the treated breast becomes slightly smaller or larger than the other one and is firmer. This is caused by fluid retention or scar tissue in the breast. Although not harmful, this can be uncomfortable.

# Recovery and reconstruction

How your breasts look after the surgery will depend on their shape and size to start with, the site of the lump, whether you have had a lumpectomy or a mastectomy and how much tissue was removed.

- After a mastectomy, the incision line will usually extend horizontally across your chest. At first this will be red, but the scar will gradually fade, though it will never be completely invisible.

- After a lumpectomy, the appearance of your breast may be little changed. There is likely to be a small scar and sometimes a small dent. If more tissue was removed you're likely to have a larger scar. Your breast will also look smaller and less full, especially if you have small breasts. The removal of breast tissue may affect the position of your nipple.

The surgeon or breast care nurse may be able to show you photos of women who have had breast surgery so that you know what to expect. Immediately after your operation, the wound will be covered with protective dressing and one or more drainage tubes to drain off blood and other fluids might be in place (although very few surgeons will insert drainage tubes after a lumpectomy). There is not usually much bleeding, especially after a lumpectomy, and if you have any drains, these will be removed after a day or so.

### When am I likely to know the results of my surgery?

Usually your surgeon will tell you how the operation itself went later on the same day or the next morning. The tissue removed will be sent to the laboratory to be examined under a microscope and analysed. As detailed analysis is required, the results usually take up to 10 days to become available, in which case you will probably be asked to visit the outpatients department to collect your results – often at the same time as you have your surgical wound checked for healing. If this is the case, it can be a good idea to take a relative or friend along with you to your appointment to help you absorb any information you are given.

## Questions to ask the doctor

- Has the cancer been completely removed?
- Am I likely to need more surgery?
- Has the cancer spread to the lymph nodes?
- Have any additional tests been carried out? If so, what are the results of these?
- Is the cancer hormone or HER-2 receptor positive? (See p.95).
- What further treatment do you recommend on the basis of the findings?

## What are the after-effects of surgery?

The precise after-effects will vary depending on different factors such as your age and state of health, your individual pain threshold, how quickly your skin heals and your feelings about surgery. However, many women feel well enough to get up the same day and most are up by the following day. Some after-effects you may experience include:

**Swelling:** Some swelling in the breast, chest wall or shoulder as the body heals itself is usual. This should normally disappear after six to eight weeks.

- Wearing a supportive bra both day and night may help ease discomfort.
- If swelling persists, you should seek advice from your breast care nurse or consultant.

**Pain and soreness:** Immediately after surgery the area operated on may be bruised and feel rather sore and tender. However, many women are surprised by how little pain they experience. Obviously the larger the operation, the more painful it is likely to be. If lymph nodes have been removed, you may feel pain and a burning discomfort in your armpit and down your inner arm. Post-operative pain will usually disappear gradually over the next six to eight weeks.

- Taking a simple painkiller like paracetamol or ibuprofen will usually sort out any problems with pain, although some women need stronger painkillers.
- If you continue to feel pain, the breast care nurse or consultant may be able to refer you to a pain specialist for help and advice.

**Stiffness:** You may experience stiffness in the arm and/or shoulder on the side operated upon, especially if you have had a mastectomy.

- The physiotherapist will see you while you're in hospital to recommend exercises for shoulder mobilisation.
- Once the dressing has been removed and the stitches taken out, the breast care nurse or physiotherapist can show you further exercises to help you regain range of movement.

**Changed sensation:** It is common after mastectomy or axillary surgery to experience a loss or change of sensation in the chest, under your arms and/or running down the inside of the upper arm as a result of nerves being cut or disturbed during the operation. Sensations may include numbness, coldness, burning, pins and needles, weakness and sensitivity to touch or pressure as a result of nerve damage. These sensations generally improve and may disappear completely over the next couple of months or so following surgery. However, some women experience permanent changed or lost sensation.

- If sensation loss is disturbing, treatments are available, so mention it to your breast care nurse or make an appointment to see the doctor.

### How am I likely to feel after axillary surgery?

At first the area can be quite painful and you may find it difficult to move your arm and/or shoulder. In general, the more lymph nodes removed the more acute the side-effects.

### How am I likely to feel emotionally after surgery?

Immediately after you come round you are likely to feel groggy and possibly nauseous due to the effects of the anaesthetic. Once you begin to recover, you may feel tired – in some cases this may last for several weeks or months. This is partly due to the after-effects of the operation and partly a result of the emotional effects of diagnosis and treatment. Some women feel a sense of relief immediately after the operation that gives them a surge of energy, only to discover that fatigue catches up with them a day or two later or when they get home. It is important to give yourself time to recover physically and emotionally.

Before your operation you may have had little time to think about anything much other than treatment. Once surgery is over, however, the full impact of your diagnosis and its implications may hit you, and you may feel a welter of different, often conflicting, emotions. You may get all the support you need from family and friends. However, some women feel they do not want to burden those close to them with their feelings. Not everyone wants help in dealing with their emotions, but if you are finding your feelings difficult to deal with it can help to talk them through with a breast care nurse. You may also find it helpful to talk to other women who have been through the same experience, either one to one or in a group. There may be a support group at the hospital where you are being treated. Alternatively, you may want to contact one of the cancer organisations listed on pages 259–60 to find out about what support is available in your area.

### What sort of pain control is available?

Simple painkillers like paracetamol or ibuprofen are often sufficient to keep any pain under control. If they aren't sufficient, you can ask for something stronger. One technique uses a long-acting local anaesthetic block, administered during the operation. This means that few, if any, painkillers will be necessary and you can remain pain-free for 24 to 36 hours.

### Should I have a reconstruction?

If you have had a mastectomy or a lumpectomy in which a more substantial area of tissue has been removed, you may be offered a reconstruction, to 'rebuild' your breast surgically. This is done either by placing an implant underneath the skin and muscle of your chest wall, by using tissue from another area of your body (autologous) or by using a combination of the two. There are advantages and disadvantages to reconstruction that you will want to consider carefully before going ahead.

**Reconstruction pros & cons**

**Pros**

- Reconstruction can help you feel more 'whole' and help to restore self-esteem and body image following mastectomy.
- Having a more natural-looking breast shape can prevent you from constantly being reminded that you have had breast cancer.
- You may feel less embarrassed in changing rooms and other places where you have to undress in public.
- You may feel more comfortable with or without clothes.

# Marja Bego

My breast cancer was picked up on my first scan, when I was 51; there was no lump. I had to wait a couple of weeks for the results, but I instinctively knew. They said it was small, so my chance of surviving was better than most. I had a lumpectomy on my left side. They seemed to think that if it was a small amount of cancer you weren't going to have much trouble but I found that I was much more physically affected than I thought I would be: fatigue, memory loss, lack of concentration. Some of us had taken books into hospital thinking: 'A week in hospital, put your feet up!' It was just a joke; we couldn't even concentrate long enough to read a page of *Woman's Weekly*. This seemed very different to other anaesthetics I'd had. Then a girl from one of the side wards worked out what it was: the painkillers. The painkillers had turned us into zombies – it just never occurred to me. We stopped taking them. I'd rather have a little bit of pain. It wasn't just the painkillers though. Irrespective of them I found my energy levels had been severely reduced – even to this day, although there has been a steady improvement. Up to a point we were warned about this. The staff said several times that from now on we would be needing frequent 'fuel stops' and this has proven to be the case. But I don't think many of us were prepared for how severe these were to be at first.

A few weeks after my surgery we went back to the hospital to see the surgeon, because when they take the tumour out they test it and they go under your arm to see if there's anything there. And they never let on that the cut under the arm was the worst. You can't sleep; you can't lie. By week five I hadn't had a proper night's sleep so I was feeling a bit miserable, and the surgeon came into the room and said 'It's good news – there's nothing there!' And I could see we were meant to be pleased, but I was just thinking: 'After all this!' And I could see Gordon was too. So I said thank you, and we didn't know whether to laugh or cry, but the side of my mouth started twitching, and I didn't want to hurt her feelings, so we just stayed neutral and left. I had to go to the loo and Gordon was waiting for me and she came up to him and said, 'Will you go out and celebrate?' and he said, 'No, we're going to B&Q.'

When I first had it done I couldn't walk because of the bouncing, the jarring. I had to walk so slowly, with my arm folded across myself to support my breast – I felt like an old lady. I had a lot of fluid retention as well, which was just a bit of a pain.

And I hated my breast when I saw it. I mean, I've done a little bit of nursing, so I know a neat scar when I see one, and it's not bad, and the nurse said, 'it's a lovely scar' and I didn't want to show how upset I was, so I just kept looking happy, but inside I just thought ooohhhh. You become so down to earth because your body image is so attacked. You see life as pre- and post-cancer – and for most of us pre-cancer is a distant light at the other end of the tunnel.

I didn't realise it would take so long to get back to normal – I found this thing on the Web and it said '1 to 2 years' and I thought, eh? But when I really sat down and thought I realised that I wasn't going to be able to continue with my course and I thought about how long I would need, and decided to ask for six months. And I went to see my tutor, and he said 'Take the year,' so I did. I was reading on the Web the other day, and this German woman was saying that the hardest part for her was getting ready for nine o'clock in the morning. And I thought, 'Yes! So it's not just me!'

**Cons**

- You may not want to undergo any further operations.
- You may have other health problems that might make it inadvisable to have more surgery and anaesthesia.
- You may be concerned about potential complications.
- You may feel you will be able to adjust to a new body image without the need for reconstruction.
- You prefer to wear an external prosthesis.

## When do I need to make up my mind?

If you think you may want an immediate reconstruction, you will have to decide before having a mastectomy. This can be tough. Faced with a diagnosis of breast cancer and the prospect of treatment it can be difficult to take in all you need to in order to make an informed decision about reconstruction as well. Some women – and breast surgeons – prefer to delay making the choice until later to give you time to absorb the implications of having breast cancer. Others, despite the complicated decision-making involved, are sure they want to go ahead straightaway. If you do decide to go ahead, the surgeon should ensure that you have time for thorough consideration of all the options before you have your operation.

## What can I expect from a reconstruction?

An important factor in how pleased you will feel with the results of reconstruction is having a realistic idea of what can be achieved. It is never possible to replace the breast you have lost. Breast reconstruction is not the same as having breast implants or breast reduction as a cosmetic procedure, although some women do take the opportunity to go for larger or smaller breasts and have surgery on the other side to achieve a balance. What reconstruction can do is provide you with a mound that mimics as far as possible your lost breast in shape, size and volume and looks like the real thing under clothes, including bras and swimwear. If you are of childbearing age and subsequently go on to have a baby, it will be impossible to breastfeed on the reconstructed side because of the absence of breast tissue, although you can still feed with the other breast. Bear in mind too that implants do tend to form capsules that harden over time so you may need to have further surgery at a later date to replace them.

It is vital to discuss these issues thoroughly with your surgeon before going ahead so that you are sure that you know exactly what to expect and have a clear idea of what the final result is likely to look like. Having said this, most women who have a reconstruction feel extremely pleased with their 'new' breast.

## Will my reconstructed breast feel the same as my other breast?

If you opt for the implant method of reconstruction, your 'new' breast will have the same weight and consistency of natural breast tissue and the skin over the reconstructed breast will feel normal to the touch because it is your skin. However, it may be harder and firmer and is usually less droopy than your natural breast. Opting for one of the techniques that utilises your own body tissue may feel more natural, although you won't have the same sensation in your reconstructed breast as in your natural breast, and it is common to have an area of skin without any sensation at all.

## Will the reconstructed breast look the same as my natural breast?

Your surgeon will do his or her best to match your natural breast and achieve a symmetrical appearance, especially when you are wearing a bra, although the nipple will usually have been removed during surgery, so prosthetic options for this may need to be considered. Without a bra your own natural breast is likely to be droopier than the reconstructed one, especially if you opt for an implant. It is possible to have your natural breast enlarged, reduced or uplifted to achieve a more symmetrical outline.

## How many operations am I likely to need?

It is important to recognise that reconstruction is a process rather than a one-off procedure. In all but the simplest cases, it is likely to involve one main operation to produce the breast mound and then a series of minor adjustments to achieve a good cosmetic result. Several operations may therefore be required over time. Additional surgery may be performed to add a nipple or to change the shape or size of the reconstructed breast.

## When might reconstruction be carried out?

Reconstruction can be carried out either at the same time as your mastectomy or lumpectomy or some months – or even years – later. As techniques improve, an increasing number of women are opting for immediate reconstruction. However, each option has its advantages and disadvantages, so it is a question of weighing up what is likely to be best for you. You should have plenty of time to discuss all the various options with the surgeon before your mastectomy or lumpectomy, although of course you don't have to come to a firm decision at this stage if you don't want to. If you are having radiotherapy, you will usually have to wait until your skin and breast have recovered from its effects before going ahead with a full reconstruction, although certain preliminary procedures may be possible beforehand.

### Immediate vs delayed reconstruction
#### Immediate
**Pros**

- Gets a large part of the surgery over and done with in one go.
- Can give women the opportunity to have a 'skin conserving' mastectomy, using a smaller incision in which the surgeon leaves an 'envelope' of skin into which an implant can be inserted (see below).
- Feelings of mutilation sometimes felt by women who have had a mastectomy or lost a lot of breast tissue may be less.
- Feelings of loss of attractiveness and femininity may be less.
- Self-esteem and confidence may be less damaged.

**Cons**

- Physical stress of having large amount of surgery at same time.
- May not be a viable alternative for all women.
- Radiotherapy is being used more and more frequently as an adjunct to mastectomy and often the decision to give radiotherapy depends on the results of the analysis of the removed breast and lymph glands. It may therefore be possible that a reconstruction procedure carried out before this information is available will compromise the quality of the result. For example, it would be unfortunate to rebuild the breast with a Latissimus Dorsi flap which was then irradiated,

preventing it stretching, whereas if a delayed reconstruction was performed then the non-irradiated Latissimus flap could be brought in to improve the irradiated tissue.

**Delayed**

**Pros**

- More time to recover from mastectomy and other treatment.
- More time to think about what you really want. Some women find losing a breast less distressing than they imagined and change their minds about reconstruction.

**Cons**

- More distress over mastectomy.
- More stress while waiting to be operated upon.
- There may be a long wait because of a shortage of surgeons experienced in delayed breast reconstruction.
- Need for a second operation and general anaesthetic.

### Who will perform my reconstruction?

There are several different options:

- A general plastic (cosmetic) surgeon – i.e. one who doesn't specialise exclusively in breast reconstruction.
- A plastic surgeon who specialises solely in reconstructive breast surgery.
- An oncological specialist breast surgeon – usually the one who performed the mastectomy.

A new speciality of oncoplastic surgery is emerging, in which one surgeon is a specialist in both breast cancer surgery and reconstruction. Currently there are not many oncoplastic surgeons in the UK. However, the Government has recently instituted a new training scheme, so there are likely to be more in the future.

The importance of getting a reputable surgeon who is experienced in carrying out the type of reconstruction that you are planning to have cannot be overemphasised. Your breast cancer specialist or breast care nurse may be able to recommend a surgeon in the same hospital or in your Health Authority area. Before you make an appointment, it might be a good idea to ask your GP about the surgeon's qualifications, experience and reputation. When you do meet the surgeon, think about how you interact with each other. It is important to feel comfortable with the person who is carrying out the operation. This is a very personal matter. If you feel at all uncomfortable, consider seeking a different surgeon or obtaining a second opinion.

**What are the different kinds of reconstruction?**
Broadly, there are three types:
- implant (saline or silicone)
- a combination of implant and the body's own tissue (usually a 'flap' of tissue is taken from the back muscle, the Latissimus Dorsi)
- using the body's own tissue alone (that is, a 'flap' of fat and skin and/or muscle from the abdomen, or sometimes from the back or buttocks)

There is no one type that is best for everyone; it is a question of tailoring the procedure to you as an individual. Some women's breasts and body form are more suited to one type of reconstruction than others. For instance, if you are slim and small-breasted, a simple implant may be the best option. If you are curvaceous and large-breasted, a TRAM implant (see p.80) using tissue from your abdomen will probably produce a better result, whereas it would be unlikely to suit a very slim woman with a flat abdomen. Your age, overall health and whether or not you smoke come into it too. If you are young, fit and in good health, you are in a better position to cope with a more complex operation (or several operations) than if you are older or unfit or have existing health problems such as diabetes or heart disease or are a smoker. All of these can affect your ability to withstand a long, complex operation, the time it takes to recover and the likelihood of complications.

You may want to discuss the various options with the surgeon, the breast care nurse and your family and/or friends. It is also important to discuss the options with other women who have chosen the same procedure and find out how it went and whether they are pleased with the result. Your surgeon or breast care nurse should be able to find someone who has been treated by your surgeon. Alternatively, organisations such as CancerBACUP, the Haven Trust and Breast Cancer Care have information booklets and may be able to put you in touch with other women who have had reconstruction.

## SIMPLE IMPLANT (subcutaneous reconstruction)

### What it is

This is very rarely done, as it involves placing an implant just under the skin and fat. More commonly done is the submuscular reconstruction (see below).

### When it might be done

If your skin and nipple have been preserved in a mastectomy or lumpectomy. Best if your breasts are not large and you do not have ptosis (droop).

### Advantages

- Discreet scar (hidden on either side and around the nipple or in the natural crease beneath the breast).
- Can give a good cosmetic result.
- A simple operation that adds little to the time or complexity of a mastectomy.
- Recovery time is little more than for a mastectomy so only a short hospital stay is required.

### Disadvantages

- Fibrous scar tissue attaching to the implant and making it hard and painful (capsular contracture) is common. In this case another operation may need to be performed to remove and replace the implant.
- This type of reconstruction is sometimes combined with nipple preservation. Some surgeons fear small deposits of cancerous cells may remain in the preserved nipple and the area around it (areola) that may grow, although the chances are small and are less if your operation is performed by a specialist.

## SUBMUSCULAR RECONSTRUCTION

### What it is

This is the most common type of reconstruction whereby an implant (a silicone shell) filled with silicone gel or saline is inserted beneath the muscle of the chest wall and skin of the breast to replace the tissue that has been removed. It is usually necessary to insert a tissue expander, which is like a small balloon and can be filled through a small port to create a pocket of a size and shape to match the other breast (see below).

## When it might be done

If you have small to moderately sized breasts and you have not had a radical mastectomy (in which case the chest muscle will have been removed, although this is rare). Not recommended if you have had radiotherapy because of the loss of skin elasticity and wound-healing problems.

## Advantages

- Straightforward operation.
- Can give a good cosmetic appearance.
- Discreet scar (in the crease of the breast or angled to the line of the mastectomy scar).

## Disadvantages

- Difficult to achieve symmetry if you have larger breasts or ptosis.
- Implant may move or change shape slightly as muscle over it contracts.
- Risk of capsular contracture as above.

## TISSUE EXPANSION

### What it is

A method of stretching the skin of the chest sufficiently to accommodate an implant. This is done over a period of months and can be done immediately after a mastectomy or as a delayed procedure. There are two types:

- A permanent silicone implant with an inflatable inner chamber is used. This is inflated over a period of weeks and left over-inflated for several weeks more. It is then deflated to a size matching your other breast. So that it cannot be felt, the valve is then removed or repositioned, under local anaesthetic.
- An operation is done to insert an expandable bag under the chest muscle. Over a period of months this bag is gently expanded by injecting a sterile saline solution through a valve to form a new breast slightly larger than the other one. The bag is then removed and another operation performed to insert a permanent implant under the expanded muscle and skin.

### When it might be done

Suitable for most women who want it, unless you have had radical mastectomy or radiotherapy, in which case the skin tissue may have lost too much elasticity to stretch sufficiently.

### Advantages

- Can give good cosmetic results.
- Makes use of skin's natural elasticity.
- Gentle, gradual method.

### Disadvantages

- You need to attend the hospital outpatient department several times following surgery for the inflation to be done.
- Slight discomfort when the breast is being expanded.
- Not suitable for all women.
- Risk of capsular contracture.

## USING AN IMPLANT AND THE BODY'S OWN TISSUE (L-D flap)

### What it is

A flap or a portion of skin, muscle and fat is taken from one part of the body and moved to the chest area, where it is formed into a mound together with an implant. Usually the large back muscle (the Latissimus Dorsi) is used because its blood supply comes from the axilla (armpit), as does that for your natural breast tissue. The whole muscle is brought around to the chest and positioned into the envelope of breast skin. Because the main blood vessels are not cut, the muscle remains healthy and protects the implant placed beneath it. A section of skin will be taken from the back over the muscle to replace the skin removed during the mastectomy. This does leave a scar on your back. Because the nerve supply to this skin will have been disrupted, it will remain numb.

### When it might be done

If tissue expansion has been tried but was unsuccessful, or if tissue expansion cannot be performed because too much skin and muscle was removed from the breast in the mastectomy. It is also suitable for women who have had radiotherapy and whose skin is not elastic enough for tissue expansion and women with small to medium or large breasts. It can be done immediately or as a delayed procedure.

### Advantages

- Suitable for women who have had radical mastectomy and/or radiotherapy.
- The tissue used is well supplied with blood vessels and usually heals well.

**Disadvantages**

- This type of reconstruction adds to operating time – usually two to three hours longer than a straightforward mastectomy.
- Recovery time is longer and involves a hospital stay of up to a week.
- Greater risk of post-operative complications such as fluid build-up (seroma) that will need to be drained (usually on a weekly basis for three to four weeks).
- You will have a scar on your back (the surgeon will usually place this beneath your bra line, so you can still wear low-cut clothes).
- If there is a poor blood supply to the flap tissue, part or all of the tissue in the breast area may not survive.

## USING THE BODY'S OWN TISSUE ALONE

**What it is**

There are four kinds:

- **TRAM flap** (Transverse Rectus Abdominis Muscle) in which skin, muscle and fat from the lower abdomen is tunnelled up to the chest area to create the new breast, allowing you to have a 'tummy tuck' as well as reconstructive breast surgery. However, the scar is bigger than in a normal 'tummy tuck' and the results not as good. The tissue creates a convincing soft breast that mimics the natural breast of a mature woman better than an implant. The biggest disadvantage is that, because muscle tissue is taken, the abdominal wall is weakened, posing a subsequent risk of abdominal hernia. Synthetic mesh may therefore be used to reinforce the abdominal wall. There is also a risk of some of the fat of the flap dying because of poor blood supply to the flap tissue; this can also result in part or all of the skin dying. There is also a risk of unsightly abdominal scarring.
- **Free TRAM flap.** TRAM flaps can be used to re-create the breast in two ways. The blood supply to the transferred tissue can be left intact on its blood vessel attached to the muscle – the pedicled flap. The TRAM flap may also be deliberately detached from its existing blood supply and reconnected, using the vessels that come from the upper end of the abdomen and joining them by microscope to vessels either from under the breast bone or from the armpit – the free TRAM flap. The free TRAM flap may

minimise muscle disruption at the donor site. The procedure is more complicated, involving microsurgery, takes longer and can often require a period in the Intensive Care Unit post-operatively, but may achieve a better blood supply to the transferred tissue.

- **DIEP** (Deep Inferior Epigastric Perforator). This is a newer technique in which skin and fat, but not muscle, is taken from the lower abdomen and left attached to blood vessels. This reduces the risk of fat necrosis (death), and because muscle is not taken the abdominal wall is not weakened, so the risk of hernia is reduced. Recovery is usually quicker, although the abdominal scar is the same as that from a TRAM flap.
- **Extended LD flap.** The tissue is taken from the same area of the back as the standard LD flap, but the skin and deeper tissues removed are more extensive, so that small and medium-sized breasts may be reconstructed without the need for an implant.

## Advantages

- Creation of a natural-looking, soft breast that is more similar to your own than a reconstruction with a breast implant.
- No risk of rejection as your own body tissue is used.
- No risk of infection of implant.
- Although numb, the tissues feel more 'normal' because they are your own.
- With an Extended LD flap, there is no abdominal scarring.

## Disadvantages

- Need for a long, complex operation.
- Longer recovery time because the surgery is complicated.
- Abdominal scarring (not with an Extended LD flap).
- Not suitable if you are contemplating a future pregnancy (still possible with a DIEP flap).
- Small risk of hernia with TRAM.
- Failure of blood supply to the transferred tissue may result in its partial or total loss.
- Partial failure of the blood supply may result in hard lumps on the reconstructed breast (fat necrosis).

Another type of tissue transfer uses tissue from the buttocks. However, it is not widely done. New techniques are constantly being developed so it is worth asking your surgeon to explain what is currently available and what their expertise in these is.

## Can I keep my nipples?

It is occasionally possible to keep your nipple if you are having immediate reconstruction, provided the surgeon thinks there is no danger that the nipple or any attached tissue contains cancer cells. The nipple is grafted onto the reconstructed breast, although this will not always happen immediately. It may be possible to graft the nipple to another part of your body until you have the reconstruction and then attach it to the new breast. Although for most patients it is not possible to keep your natural nipple, nipple reconstruction is possible at a later date, using grafted skin tissue from elsewhere on your body or a tattoo. Silicone stick-on nipples are also available.

## Will I be in pain?

Any kind of surgery will usually involve pain. However, some women say they were surprised by the fact that the pain lasts for several months after reconstructive surgery. The amount of pain varies considerably, and will depend on the type of operation you had for your breast cancer and whether lymph glands were removed, as well as your personal pain threshold. If you are finding pain particularly troublesome, tell your doctor or breast care nurse as there are many effective techniques for pain control – techniques to control post-operative pain are well established and are very effective.

## Are there any potential complications?

Any kind of surgery carries a risk of complications. These will be similar to those already described, such as risk of infection (which can sometimes mean removing an implant), pain, swelling, bruising, tenderness and scarring (see p.67). These will disappear as your body heals and the scars will fade gradually. There are a few complications specific to reconstruction. These include:

- **Capsular contracture**, caused by fibrous scar tissue forming around an implant causing tightening, hardening and changes in the shape of the reconstructed breast. Improvements in technique and implants have led to fewer cases. However, in a few instances, the implant and capsule may have to be removed and a new implant put in.

- **Asymmetry.** As far as possible the surgeon will try to create a breast that matches your natural breast. However, sometimes there is a degree of asymmetry (uneven appearance). Losing or putting on weight can sometimes help. Alternatively, it may be possible to have surgery on your other breast to create a more even appearance.
- **Muscle weakness** in the area where a skin flap was taken from can be a problem, causing abdominal hernia or shoulder and/or arm weakness.
- **Poor healing.** If you are a smoker, a diabetic or obese, you may heal less well after surgery because of a poorer blood supply to the tissues.
- **Seroma** (see p.57), especially in the back donor site after a Latissimus reconstruction (see p.79).

## If I decide to have an implant, is silicone safe?

Concerns about silicone stem back to the 1990s, when a number of women in the US claimed that silicone implants had caused them to develop connective tissue disorders and autoimmune problems such as scleroderma, rheumatoid arthritis and fibromyalgia. Since then, a large number of scientific studies have been done showing that silicone is safe. There is no evidence that silicone implants cause cancer or delay subsequent detection or recurrence of breast cancer. When any 'foreign body' enters the body, there is a risk of infection and rejection. For this reason, you will have a course of antibiotics to prevent infection. However, if it is a problem, the implant may have to be removed. Usually, another one can be inserted in a few months time.

## Questions to ask your doctor

- How many reconstructions have you done/do you do each year? Experts estimate that slightly less than 40 per cent of women in a unit will normally have a mastectomy. The key factor is what percentage of those having a mastectomy and who opt for reconstruction the surgeon sees – look for a surgeon who is performing about 20–40 per cent of these reconstructions. Also find out what kinds of procedures the surgeon performs, and how many of each type. More than 25 per year is desirable.

- Can you show me photos of breast reconstructions you have done? Ask to see both best and worst results.
- What type of surgery do you recommend for me and why?
- Can you put me in touch with other women who have had this type of reconstruction?
- How long will the operation take?
- What kind of anaesthesia will be used?
- What is current medical thinking about breast implant safety?
- When do you recommend I should begin having my breast reconstructed?
- How many operations am I likely to need?
- How can I expect my breast to look and feel after surgery?
- What are the long-term effects likely to be?
- Will I have scars? If so, where will they be situated and how large are they likely to be?
- If I opt for flap surgery, will there be permanent changes where the tissue was removed?
- Are there likely to be any complications? What percentage of women you operate on develop complications?
- How long will I need to stay in hospital?
- How long will it take me to recover?
- When can I return to my normal activities?
- Are there any activities I should avoid?
- What follow-up care is likely to be needed?

**What if I don't like the results?**

How happy you will feel with the reconstruction is closely related to your expectations. That is why it is important to discuss your options and understand what you can realistically expect before going ahead. It will usually take several months for the reconstructed breast to begin to look and feel normal. If you are still unhappy after that, make an appointment to see the surgeon or the breast care nurse.

**Could a breast implant mask a recurrence of cancer?**

Experts consider that there is little or no risk of not detecting a recurrent cancer after a mastectomy. If cancer does recur, it will usually do so just under the skin and should be easily detectable by palpation (feeling).

## If I decide not to opt for reconstruction, what are my alternatives?

If you decide reconstruction is not for you, or have chosen to delay having reconstruction, you can use an external breast prosthesis, an artificial breast form made from silicone gel, that fits into your bra. Prostheses are available in different shapes, sizes and skin colours. Many include a nipple outline, or you may choose to have a false nipple that you stick on to the prosthesis. It is also possible to have a nipple custom-made to match the one on your other breast.

The most common prosthesis is put inside your bra and sits snugly against your chest wall. Other types include:

### PARTIAL PROSTHESIS

**What it is**

Either a hollow 'shell' that fits over your remaining breast tissue creating a more rounded shape, or a crescent of silicone that fills out the bottom, side or top of your bra.

**Who it's for**

If you have had a lumpectomy and have lost enough breast tissue for your breast shape to have been affected.

### LIGHTWEIGHT PROSTHESIS

**What it is**

Silicone prosthesis that weighs less than your normal breast or a normal weight prosthesis.

**Who it's for**

If you feel that a normal weight prosthesis is too heavy for you.

### SELF-SUPPORTING PROSTHESIS

**What it is**

A prosthesis that can be stuck onto your skin either directly or using adhesive tape.

**Who it's for**

If you are concerned about the prosthesis slipping out of your bra, or you do a lot of sports or other physical activities.

## Where can I be fitted for a prosthesis?

The breast care nurse may fit you, or in many breast units there is a special appliance officer. Breast Cancer Care has a free fitting service in London, Glasgow and Edinburgh. For an appointment, telephone 020 7384 2984 (London) or 0141 221 2244 (Glasgow and Edinburgh). Prostheses obtained through the NHS are available free. Alternatively, you can buy them through mail order suppliers and from some high street stores. Expect to pay from around £85. VAT is exempt if you have had surgery for breast cancer.

## How soon can I have a prosthesis?

You will usually be able to wear a prosthesis after your scar has healed (around six to eight weeks after surgery) and after you have had any radiotherapy, as your skin is likely to be tender and sensitive for a while. A soft prosthesis (a 'comfy') is offered soon after surgery, before discharge from hospital. This is a light prosthesis made of synthetic washable fibre inside a cotton cover to tide you over until you are able to have an external silicone one.

## Will I have to pay for a prosthesis?

If you had your surgery on the NHS, you can choose a prosthesis free. This can be replaced free of charge when it shows signs of wear, is damaged, or if you gain or lose a lot of weight. If you were treated through a private healthcare scheme, you'll need to check your policy to see if it covers the cost of your prosthesis.

# Adjuvant treatment

Adjuvant treatment, sometimes called adjuvant therapy, is the treatment that is given in addition to a primary therapy. For breast cancer, surgery is usually the primary therapy, with chemotherapy, hormone treatment or radiotherapy given as additional or adjuvant treatment. (See p.63 for details of radiotherapy).

**What is chemotherapy and when is it used?**

Chemotherapy is treatment with cytotoxic (cancer-killing) drugs. It is used for three main reasons:

- to prevent recurrence after primary local treatment to the breast
- as the main treatment for advanced cancer
- to relieve symptoms in cancer that has spread to other parts of the body

Adjuvant chemotherapy is designed to prevent recurrence by destroying cancer cells that may have spread from the breast to other parts of the body which could, left untreated, develop into cancers.

**Why is the doctor recommending chemotherapy when I've just had surgery to remove the cancer?**

Malignant tumours are made up of millions of cells that are capable of travelling from the breast to other parts of the body, a process known as metastasis. When only a few cancer cells have spread from the breast (micrometastases), they can elude detection by standard tests and scans. Therefore it is important to eradicate them to try to prevent them from developing into secondary tumours elsewhere in the body. The doctor will base the decision to recommend chemotherapy on the likelihood or level of risk that cancer cells may already have spread, or may do so at some time in the future.

**Will chemotherapy prevent my cancer from recurring?**

Although the aim of chemotherapy is to reduce the risk of recurrence, no treatment is guaranteed to prevent future cancers. Research has shown that chemotherapy significantly decreases the odds of cancer recurring and may prevent it altogether.

**What factors will the doctor take into account when recommending chemotherapy?**

Because your doctors cannot predict with absolute certainty whether your breast cancer is likely to return or spread, they will make a careful assessment based on the risks versus the benefits for you. This will include:

- **The risk of recurrence:** how likely it is that your cancer will recur in your particular case.
- **The benefit of chemotherapy:** how much the doctor thinks chemotherapy will help you and by how much it will reduce the risk of recurrence.
- **Side-effects:** how chemotherapy is likely to affect you and what short- and long-term side-effects it is likely to have.

In weighing up your personal risk/benefit equation the doctor will consider:

- **Your age:** cancers in younger women may be more aggressive and so are more likely to be treated with chemotherapy.
- **The size of your tumour:** usually you will be offered chemotherapy if the tumour was larger than 2 cm in diameter.
- **Whether cancer cells have been found in the axillary nodes:** This is the single most important factor in whether cancer is likely to recur.
- **The appearance of the cancer cells under a microscope:** This is called the grade of the tumour, and is based on the shape and size of the cells and whether they are dividing rapidly (see p.37).
- **The hormonal status of the tumour:** whether it has receptors onto which hormones can lock that encourage it to grow (see p.95).

**How can I decide whether I might benefit from chemotherapy?**

In some cases the indications are fairly clear. For example, if you are under 50 and in good health with a node-positive, fast-growing cancer, chemotherapy is likely to offer you the best chance of remaining cancer free. In this case you may feel that you are prepared to put up with potential side-effects and disruption to your life. In other instances it can be more difficult, for example, if you are older and have a small, slow-growing cancer, if you are unfit or have other medical conditions that may make it more difficult to deal with side-effects. Your doctor should give you facts and figures about remission rates and the likelihood of relapse based on the available evidence. However, bear in mind that this evidence is changing all the time as new trials are conducted, as new drugs and drug combinations become available and as researchers learn more about breast cancer. Only you, together with your doctor, can decide what impact chemotherapy is likely to have on your life. Take time to discuss the relative costs and benefits with your doctor or breast care nurse and seek further information from one of the cancer organisations (see pages 259–60) if you need to.

### Questions to ask your doctor

- Is chemotherapy usually recommended for my particular kind of breast cancer?
- Why are you recommending chemotherapy for me at this time?
- Are there any other options?
- What is the chance of recurrence if I go ahead?
- How many courses of chemotherapy am I likely to need?
- How long will treatment last?
- What drugs will be used?
- How will the drugs be administered?
- How will you know if it's working?
- What side-effects can I expect? (See p.91)

### Will I have to wait for chemotherapy?

Chemotherapy is usually given after surgery and before any radiotherapy. Treatment will usually begin two to four weeks following surgery (although anything up to eight weeks is acceptable) to allow your body the chance to recover from the operation. If you do have to wait, bear in mind that adjuvant chemotherapy is essentially precautionary rather than urgent, so although waiting is not ideal, it should not affect your long-term outlook.

### My specialist has recommended a course of chemotherapy before surgery. Why?

Sometimes a tumour is too large to perform surgery, and sometimes the risk of local recurrence in the chest wall is high – for example, if you have a fast-growing, inflammatory cancer. In these circumstances, the doctor may recommend a course of chemotherapy – usually lasting from three to six months – to shrink the tumour and make surgery possible. This is called neoadjuvant or primary chemotherapy. One advantage of giving chemotherapy first is that it may reduce the size of a lump sufficiently to make it possible for you to have a lumpectomy rather than mastectomy. It can also help your doctor to assess how sensitive the cancer cells are to drug treatment, which can help in planning future treatment.

**If chemotherapy is given first, will I still need surgery?**
Even after chemotherapy the surgeon will always remove the area where the breast cancer was, because in most cases there is microscopic evidence of cancer. Although there are no residual cells after primary chemotherapy in some cases, doctors cannot, as yet, identify these women. In years to come, however, with better anti-cancer drugs, there is a distinct possibility that some women with breast cancer might not need surgery at all.

**How is chemotherapy administered?**
Chemotherapy drugs are administered in several ways:
- orally in tablet or capsule form
- by intravenous injection (injection into a vein)
- by a drip (infusion)
- by being pumped directly into your body through a tube known as a Hickman line using a battery-operated portable pump

The drugs are given in courses lasting anything from a day or less to a few days followed by a rest period of three to four weeks to allow your body to recover. The exact number of courses you will need depends on the nature of your cancer and how well it responds to treatment.

**What drugs will I have to take, and how many?**
You will almost always be prescribed a combination of two or more chemotherapy drugs (polychemotherapy). Research has found that this is the most effective way of keeping cancer at bay and also helps to reduce the effects on normal cells. There is a range of chemotherapy drugs available. The doctor can talk you through the ones recommended for you and explain why they have chosen them. You may also want to investigate the drugs prescribed yourself by checking a cancer charity website such as CancerBACUP.

### Will I have to go into hospital again?

Chemotherapy is usually administered in the outpatients department by a specialist cancer nurse. In some instances you may have to spend a few days in hospital so that the doctor can decide on the optimum dose and observe how you respond and how the drugs affect you.

### Will I be able to live a normal life while having chemotherapy?

This will depend on your individual lifestyle, your overall state of health, the drugs prescribed and how you respond to them. You will, of course, have to make time for hospital visits – usually about half a day including waiting time and treatment: it may be possible to schedule these so that there is the least possible disruption to your life. Most people having chemotherapy find it tiring but many feel well enough to continue with their normal lives with a few adjustments. The doctor should be able to tell you when the greatest fatigue and/or other side-effects are most likely to strike so as to help you organise your schedule.

### What side-effects can I expect?

As well as killing cancer cells, chemotherapy drugs may also kill some normal cells and it is this that is responsible for its side-effects. The most visible and often the most distressing is hair loss. Other side-effects include nausea, vomiting, susceptibility to infections, sore mouth, mouth ulcers, anaemia and fatigue. The doctor can give you some idea of what side-effects you might expect from the drugs you have been prescribed. However, it can be hard to predict in advance exactly how chemotherapy will affect any individual as the effects can vary wildly, even between people taking the same drugs. Although side-effects are usually the most unpleasant aspect of chemotherapy, there are many ways to manage them, so don't suffer in silence. The chemotherapy nurse and/or doctor will be able to advise you on measures that can help.

### Questions to ask your doctor

- What short-term side-effects might I experience?
- What long-term side-effects might I experience?
- How serious are these likely to be?
- How long are side-effects likely to last?

- Is there anything I can do to alleviate side-effects?
- When do you need to know about side-effects?

## Dealing with side-effects:
### Hair loss
- Ask the breast care nurse or doctor about 'scalp cooling'. This involves having an ice pack or special cold cap on your head while the drug is being given. This constricts blood vessels in the scalp, preventing the drug from reaching the hair roots and thus reducing damage to or loss of hair.
- Look after your hair carefully while you are having treatment and avoid perms, relaxing treatments, colourants and other harsh products.
- Experiment with hats, scarves and/or wigs. You may be entitled to a wig free on the NHS. Ask the breast care nurse or doctor.
- If you do lose your hair, it will grow back over a period of three to six months, although it may be a different texture or colour.

### Sore mouth
- Clean teeth with a soft toothbrush after meals.
- Use mouthwashes to discourage bacteria.
- Avoid spicy or acidic foods.
- If eating is difficult, try meal replacement drinks and shakes.

### Anaemia
- Anaemia can cause breathlessness, weakness and fatigue. If you develop these, consult the doctor. You may be given iron tablets or a blood transfusion.
- Eat a well-balanced diet. Try to include iron-rich foods, such as red meat, dried apricots, green leafy vegetables and sesame seeds.
- Cut back on non-essential activities.
- Get up slowly from sitting or lying to avoid dizziness.

### Susceptibility to infection
Chemotherapy lowers the number of infection-fighting white blood cells (neutrophils) in your body, which may make you more vulnerable to infections. Your blood will be tested regularly to determine what changes occur in your white blood cells, so infection may be treated or prevented immediately with antibiotics. You should also consult your GP if you develop signs of infection such as a sore throat or raised temperature.

Other steps you can take:

- Pay particular attention to personal hygiene. Wash your hands before eating, after using the toilet and after touching animals.
- Avoid people with obvious infections such as colds.
- Avoid crowded places such as shopping centres, pubs and cinemas – try to restrict visits to less busy times.
- Check with the doctor before having any immunisations and avoid live vaccines such as the BCG injection for tuberculosis, measles, rubella (German measles), polio and yellow fever.
- Take care with food preparation and eating out to avoid food-poisoning infections.
- Avoid activities where you may be at risk of cuts and grazes.

**Nausea and vomiting**

Anti-sickness tablets are routinely given with chemotherapy and for several days after treatment. If you find yourself experiencing nausea or vomiting, you might try one or all of the following:

- Try to eat little and often rather than only having main meals.
- Keep up your fluid intake. You may find it helps to drink before or after meals rather than with a meal.
- Avoid cooking strong-smelling foods like garlic or spices which can increase nausea. Eating food cold can reduce its aroma.
- Try eating a piece of dry toast or a cracker before getting up if morning sickness is a problem. Ginger ale might also help.
- If you do get an attack of nausea, try breathing slowly and deeply. Often the sensation will pass.
- Rest after eating.
- Complementary therapies such as relaxation, hypnosis, aromatherapy or acupressure may help.

If nausea is uncontrollable, or you have been vomiting for more than one day or cannot drink fluids, consult the doctor, who should be able to prescribe different or stronger anti-nausea drugs to prevent or reduce symptoms.

**I feel I'm being pressured into having chemotherapy. Are there any alternatives?**

Your doctor may believe that chemotherapy is the best treatment for your particular kind of cancer. However, he or she can only make a recommendation. Only you can make the final choice as to whether you want to go ahead. If you decide not to have chemotherapy, there may be other treatments that can be used depending on the exact nature of your cancer (see below), although most cancer specialists believe that when chemotherapy is indicated nothing else is quite as effective, especially when the disease is in its early stages.

## What is hormone therapy and when might it be used?

Hormones are chemical messengers produced by glands of the body's endocrine system. Oestrogen is one example. Hormone (endocrine) therapy is treatment that blocks the effects of hormones on cancer cells to stop or slow their growth. It includes:

- drugs that block the way hormones (oestrogens in particular) work on cells
- surgical techniques such as oophorectomy (removal of the ovaries) to stop the production of oestrogen

Hormone therapy may be used:

- before surgery is performed to shrink a tumour (known as neoadjuvant or primary medical therapy)
- to prevent cancer recurring after surgery is performed (known as adjuvant therapy)
- to treat advanced metastatic breast cancer

Research is going on to see whether tamoxifen, the most widely used hormonal therapy, might prevent breast cancer in women at high risk (see p.19).

Tamoxifen is currently prescribed for some 70 per cent of all women diagnosed with breast cancer, following local treatment. Tamoxifen is the treatment against which all other forms of the therapy are evaluated.

## Is hormone therapy the same as hormone replacement therapy (HRT)?

Although the terms are similar, the two treatments are completely different. HRT involves replacing supplies of the female sex hormone oestrogen (and if you have not had a hysterectomy, progesterone) that drop at the menopause, in order to treat short-term symptoms such as hot flushes and vaginal dryness and to prevent long-term effects that may arise from lack of oestrogen, such as the brittle bone disease, osteoporosis. HRT is not used as a treatment for breast cancer.

In fact, new research shows that it may slightly increase the risk of developing it (see p.99). Hormonal treatments like tamoxifen work by latching onto hormone receptors (proteins found within cells that bind to different hormones), rather like a key fitting into a lock, so preventing hormones affecting the cell.

### I've been told my tumour is hormone receptor positive (ER+ve/PgR+ve). What does this mean?

All normal breast cells have receptors for the female sex hormones oestrogen and progesterone, which are produced by the ovaries. These receptors allow the hormones to act on your breast during the menstrual cycle to prepare your body for a potential pregnancy, and during pregnancy to prepare your body for breast feeding. Some breast cancer cells also have hormone receptors. If hormones produced by the glands, or by the tumour itself, latch onto these receptors, this can stimulate the growth of the tumour. Such tumours are known as being receptor positive. Tumours that are oestrogen receptor positive are termed ER+ve, from the US spelling of oestrogen (estrogen). Tumours that are progesterone positive are known as PR+ve.

### How might hormonal therapy benefit me?

Research has proved that hormone therapy can reduce the risk of breast cancer recurring, especially in women who have gone through the menopause before being diagnosed with breast cancer and also in younger women whose tumours are hormone receptor positive. One of the biggest advantages of hormone therapy is that it is very safe and rarely causes severe or serious side-effects.

### What hormonal therapies might I be offered?

This will depend on the nature of your cancer, whether you have been through the menopause and what other treatments you have had or are having. The main ones are:

### TAMOXIFEN e.g. Nolvadex, Tamofen
#### What it is and when it might be used

An anti-oestrogen drug used as adjuvant therapy following surgery and/or radiotherapy and sometimes as a treatment for secondary breast cancer. Although the role of tamoxifen is not yet fully understood, one important action is blocking oestrogen receptors within breast cancer cells, thereby starving ER+ve tumours of their stimulus to grow. However, this is clearly not the only way in which it works, as the research has suggested that some women with ER-ve tumours may sometimes respond to tamoxifen.

**What to expect**

The drug is taken daily in tablet form for a period of five years. Taking tamoxifen in this way has been found to give significant protection against breast cancer recurrence.

**Possible side-effects**

One of the many things that doctors like about tamoxifen is that it has so few side-effects, and those it does produce are generally manageable. It also has some significant benefits, including protecting against osteoporosis and heart disease. The most common short-term side-effects include menopausal symptoms such as hot flushes, night sweats, vaginal dryness, increased vaginal discharge and weight gain, all caused by the drug's anti-oestrogenic effect. In the longer term, tamoxifen can slightly increase the risk of endometrial cancer. It can also raise the risk of thrombosis in the leg (blood clot) and eye problems such as blurred vision. If you are taking tamoxifen and are due to have surgery for a reason other than your breast cancer you should inform your surgeon that you are taking it. However, it must be stressed that these side-effects are extremely rare and almost always treatable. You should report any vaginal bleeding (except normal periods) to your doctor.

**AROMATASE INHIBITORS e.g. Arimidex, Femara, Lentaron**
**What they are and when they might be used**

A group of drugs used for women who have gone through the menopause. They are most often used to treat breast cancer that has spread or metastasised, although some trials are researching use of particular aromatase inhibitors before or after surgery for breast cancer. Aromatase inhibitors work by blocking the production of oestrogen by the adrenal glands and in fatty (adipose) tissue, which continue to produce oestrogen after the menopause by converting the male hormone testosterone (made by the adrenal gland in women) into oestrogen.

**What to expect**

It is taken as a daily tablet.

**Possible side-effects**

Few side-effects. The most common are hot flushes, nausea and, rarely, joint pains.


## PROGESTOGENS e.g. Farlutal, Provera, Megace

**What they are and how they are used**

Synthetic forms of the female sex hormone progesterone, used if hormonal therapy such as tamoxifen or aromatase inhibitors have stopped being effective.

**What to expect**

They are given in tablet form.

**Possible side-effects**

Few, but may include mild nausea, increase in appetite, weight gain (especially around the abdomen), swollen legs and ankles as a result of fluid retention, 'spotting' (small amounts of vaginal bleeding), mild muscle cramps and uterine bleeding on withdrawal.


## PITUITARY DOWNREGULATORS e.g. Zoladex

**What they are and when they might be used**

A group of drugs also known as LHRH analogues (Lutenising Hormone Releasing Hormone) that stop oestrogen production temporarily by acting on the pituitary gland. They are only used in pre-menopausal women with ER+ve breast cancer. They work by blocking the production of a 'releasing' hormone, LHRH, produced by the pituitary, a small gland at the base of the brain that triggers other glands into action. This in turn reduces the level of oestrogen in the body by stopping production in the ovaries.

**What to expect**

Administered by monthly injection into the abdomen.

**Potential side-effects**

The drug induces a temporary menopause, and may cause menopausal symptoms including hot flushes, sweats, loss of libido, headaches and mood changes.

## OOPHORECTOMY AND OVARIAN ABLATION

### What they are and when they might be used

The ovaries are removed surgically (oophorectomy) or their action is switched off (ovarian ablation) using a low dose of radiotherapy. This is used for pre-menopausal women with breast cancer. By removing the body's main source of oestrogen in pre-menopausal women, most of the oestrogen supply to a breast tumour is removed (although tumours can also produce some oestrogen). This reduces the risk of recurrence and can slow the growth of cancer cells that have spread elsewhere.

### What to expect

A surgical operation or radiotherapy treatment.

### Potential side-effects

Because the treatment induces an early menopause, side-effects are menopausal symptoms such as hot flushes, sweats and vaginal dryness.

### Questions to ask your doctor

- What hormonal therapy are you suggesting and why?
- How might this benefit me?
- How safe is it?
- What short- and long-term side-effects might there be?
- How can I deal with these?
- How long will I need to continue the therapy?
- Are there any alternatives?

### What are biological therapies and am I likely to be offered them?

Biological therapies harness the body's own immune system to fight cancer. One that has received a lot of publicity is a drug known as Herceptin (trastuzumab), which is given by infusion into a vein. Around 30 per cent of women with breast cancer have tumours that possess receptors for a growth factor called HER2 that stimulates cells to divide. These tumours are known as HER2 positive tumours. Herceptin is a monoclonal antibody. It acts by latching onto HER2 receptors, thereby blocking HER2 from stimulating the growth of the cancer. It also enhances the effect of chemotherapy, and in trials has helped women who have not responded to chemotherapy.

Currently in the UK it is only used to treat women with advanced disease that has spread, and is either given alone or with a chemotherapy drug called paclitaxel (Taxol).

**Are there any side-effects?**
It can cause flu-like symptoms and rashes at the site of the injection, although this usually wears off with continued treatment. More seriously, when given with a chemotherapy drug called doxorubicin (Adriamycin), there is a risk of heart failure. It may also affect the lungs, causing breathing problems.

**Can I continue with HRT after treatment for breast cancer?**
Recent studies have shown that long-term HRT use can increase the risk of breast cancer. However, the jury is still out on whether it is safe to take HRT if you have had breast cancer. Many doctors are reluctant to prescribe hormone replacement therapy (HRT) when you have had breast cancer, as the female hormone oestrogen can stimulate cancer cells (especially ER+ve tumours) to grow. However, some research suggests that HRT may actually help in cases where tumours have become resistant to the effects of tamoxifen and the tumour has 'learnt' to live in an oestrogen-free environment. Two large trials are being conducted in the US and in the UK, but their results will not be available until 2008 and 2011 respectively.

**What are clinical trials and should I take part in one?**
Clinical trials are research studies designed to compare new treatments – or new ways of using existing treatments – with tried and tested treatments, in order to help doctors plan more effective ways of treating disease in the future. Each study tries to answer specific questions. They have been found to be the most reliable way of testing new treatments. Trials have to conform to strict protocols. This means that, if you do participate in one, your treatment and its effects will be closely monitored every step of the way. The results of each trial are carefully analysed by trained scientists before they are published. Research shows that people who take part in trials respond to their treatment better than those who don't take part. However, only 4 per cent of patients take part in trials.

**Will I be forced to take part in a trial if my doctor suggests it?**

Your participation in any trial you are offered a place on is entirely voluntary, and you should never feel as if you are being coerced into taking part. Before you consent to take part, you should be given the opportunity to discuss in full details of what the trial involves, the potential risks and benefits of the proposed treatment and what form any monitoring will take, both with your healthcare providers and with your family and friends. Feel free to ask as many questions as you want (see below) before giving your consent to enter the trial. You may want to take a family member or friend along for support when you ask your questions and to take a tape recorder or notepad on which to record the answers. If you do decide to go ahead, bear in mind that it is your right to leave the trial at any time you want.

**Pros and cons of entering a trial**

**Pros**

- Opportunity to test a new treatment that may be more effective than current ones before it is widely available.
- Close monitoring of treatment and its effects and the chance to discuss these with your healthcare provider.
- The feeling that you are taking an active part in your care.
- The knowledge you are helping people with future breast cancer.

**Cons**

- In some trials you will not know whether you are being treated with the new treatment or the standard one.
- New treatments are not necessarily better than older ones, although it is guaranteed that the treatment you will be given will be at least as effective as the standard treatment usually given.
- The new treatment may cause unanticipated side-effects.
- The treatment may not work for you, although this applies to any treatment.
- More tests and consultations than you would have if you were having standard treatment.

**Questions to ask your doctor**

- What are you trying to find out?
- Why do you think the new treatment or approach may be effective?
- Who is backing the trial?

- How long will the trial last and when will the results be available?
- Who will be in charge of my care and where will I have my care?
- If I take part, what will this involve? What medications and/or procedures will I have to undergo and how will these be administered? What tests will be performed? Will I have to keep any sort of written record or answer a questionnaire?
- How do these compare with the medications and/or procedures I would undergo with standard treatment and the kinds of tests I would have if I didn't participate in the trial?
- Will I be able to take other medications I have been prescribed while in the trial?
- What are the potential risks and benefits of the proposed new treatment – both short- and long-term?
- What other treatment options are there and how do the possible risks and benefits of this treatment compare with those?
- What effect could being in the trial have on my everyday life?
- Can I talk to other people who are taking part in the trial?
- Are there likely to be any additional travel costs involved, and are these refundable?

### Can complementary therapies help?

Because the modern medical treatment of cancer is so complex, it can sometimes feel as if your body is not your own and that it is the doctors and nurses who are treating you rather than you who is in control. Complementary therapies such as massage, relaxation and healing can help restore your sense of control and make you feel less stressed. They can:

- ease pain and anxiety
- alleviate some side-effects of medical treatments such as nausea and vomiting
- help you come to terms with your diagnosis
- in advanced cancer can help ease late effects of cancer, such as pain

Many complementary therapies have the potential to increase your sense of well-being. Sadly, what they cannot do is effect a cure. It is very important to have realistic expectations of what can and can't be achieved if you do decide to consult a complementary practitioner.

## How can I find a complementary therapist?

Although the situation is changing, complementary therapists are, as yet, largely unregulated. This means that the onus is on you to check the credentials of any therapist you consult.

- Make sure that any practitioner you consult is registered with one of the complementary therapy organisations. (See p.260)
- Check whether any practitioner you consult has indemnity insurance.
- If you do decide to use complementary therapies, your breast care nurse or GP or your cancer support group may be able to suggest a reputable practitioner.
- Avoid anyone who promises a miracle cure.

## What about dietary therapies?

An increasing amount of research suggests that fruits, vegetables and herbs contain plant chemicals that can help protect against cancer. Eating these foods as part of a healthy, balanced diet can help improve your overall health and sense of well-being. More suspect are the various diets that claim to cure cancer, such as the Gerson diet, the Hippocrates wheat grass diet or the macrobiotic diet. Much as you may want to believe in their efficacy, none of these has been scientifically proven to cure. For some women they can be stressful to follow, restrictive, unpalatable and cause unwanted weight loss.

## Are any complementary therapies available on the NHS?

Although most complementary therapies are practised by private practitioners and you will have to pay for them, several cancer centres, support groups and hospices do offer some complementary therapies. Healers are available in some cancer centres and a growing number of nurses are training in therapies such as aromatherapy or therapeutic touch. Reflexology too is increasingly available in cancer units and hospices. There are also five NHS homeopathic hospitals. Your breast care nurse should be able to tell you what is available in your hospital. Some private medical plans will fund complementary therapies.

# Getting back to normal

Whatever steps you take to start getting back to normal, your body's natural healing mechanism will kick in of its own accord. Your skin will heal, you will regain any hair you have lost (although it may be thinner or of a different texture) and you should gradually start to feel more energetic. Most women find it takes around three to six months before they regain their usual vigour, although it can take longer. Give yourself time, and don't feel discouraged if you can't always do as much as you would like. Begin with simple, easily achievable steps such as eating a healthy diet and including some light activity that you would normally enjoy, such as a daily walk in the fresh air. At the same time you can gradually begin to take on everyday activities such as housework and driving.

However tired you feel, activity will help to increase energy and help you avoid problems such as the formation of scar tissue, muscle shortening, lymphoedema and general stiffness caused by lack of use. Breast Cancer Care have suggestions for exercises to help you get started. As you begin to feel fitter you can start doing more. If you haven't previously thought too much about living a healthy lifestyle, having breast cancer may prove a turning-point and you may discover a new interest in finding ways to look after yourself physically, mentally and emotionally.

### When can I start driving again?
You should be able to drive as soon as your wound has healed and you have regained movement in your arm. The area treated can sometimes feel a bit sore or sensitive, in which case putting some padding around the seat belt can help ease pressure. Bear in mind that some chemo-therapy drugs can make you extremely tired, or even cause dizziness and confusion in some cases. Don't drive unless you feel up to it.

### When can I go back to work?
Not only is work necessary financially, it also contributes to feelings of self-esteem. Many of us define ourselves at least in part by the job we do, and continuing to work or returning to work can be an

important part of beginning to feel normal again. If you have had time off, the exact timing of your return will depend on the treatment you have had or are having, as well as on the nature of your job, how physical it is and how much stress it involves. Some employers may be willing to let you start back part-time at first. If your job involves lifting or heavy physical activity and/or if you are finding your job too demanding, it may be possible to change to something less demanding – either temporarily or permanently – until you regain your strength. As well as the practicalities of returning to work, you'll also need to consider how to deal with the reactions of colleagues and workmates. Some women feel it is part of their work persona not to divulge too much about their illness or how they are feeling. Others will want to share more. It depends both on your personality and on the environment in which you work.

**Questions to consider when returning to work**
- How physically strenuous is your job?
- How stressful is your job?
- Does your work involve long hours or overtime?
- Will it be possible to arrange to work flexible hours?
- Can you change to part-time?
- How will you deal with talking about your illness to workmates or colleagues?

To find out more about your employment rights and/or answer questions about safety and health at work, contact your breast cancer nurse, personnel officer or one of the cancer organisations.

**How can I start to adjust to coping with the loss of my breast?**
For most women, breasts have a huge personal, social and sexual significance. Your personal reaction to the loss of your breast will depend on all sorts of factors, including your personality and outlook on life, how you thought and felt about your breasts before and the reaction of people close to you like your partner, your children, other relatives and friends. No one can predict in advance how they are going to feel, and there are no rules. If your self-identity is closely tied to your breasts, you may feel what you perceive as a loss of femininity acutely. Other women may feel saddened but are able to grieve and then move on. Some women

find it helps to talk about their feelings to others – either relatives or friends, the breast care nurse or other women who have faced the same experience. Others just want to forget about the experience and get on with their lives. The key thing is to accept your feelings as your way of coping.

## Will breast cancer affect my sex life?

If and how having breast cancer affects your sex life will depend on your interest in sex, your level of sexual activity before having breast cancer, as well as how having cancer and its treatment have affected you. It is not at all unusual for the strain of having breast cancer, energy-draining treatments and possible changes in physical appearance such as a mastectomy, hair loss and weight gain to dent the desire for sex – at least temporarily. It is often said that the mind is the biggest sex organ, and it's hard to feel sexy if you are anxious, have lost a breast or your hair and are feeling tired. Having said this, by no means all women who have had breast cancer experience a downturn in their sex lives, and those who do may find that their interest returns as they regain their energy. Breast cancer treatments can cause difficulties such as a breast tenderness, soreness or loss of sensation in the affected breast. Early menopause brought on by some treatments and its consequences, such as vaginal dryness and lack of sensitivity, can also be problematic.

If you are single or not currently in a sexual partnership but would like to be in one, there are likely to be different issues to face. Will anyone ever fancy you again? How do you tell a new partner that you have had breast cancer? How will a new partner react if you have had a mastectomy? How you deal with this will depend on you and who you meet. As with any relationship, it is a question of feeling your way as you go along and applying a certain amount of trial and error. If you are in a sexual relationship, talking to your partner about how you feel as you go through treatment and beyond can help, although it's not always easy to convey the subtleties of your feelings.

- If the drugs you are taking have caused vaginal dryness, try using a lubricant such as Senselle or KY Jelly.
- Give yourself time to adjust to changes in your physical appearance. Be open with your partner about your worries – his or her reaction may be completely different to the one you imagine.

- If penetrative sex is impossible, or if you simply do not feel like it for the time being, stroking, kissing and caressing can help you and your partner feel closer.
- Your doctor, breast care nurse or CancerBACUP counsellor can help talk you through any concerns you may have.
- Bear in mind that problems with sex are common – they will usually become easier to deal with as you recover.

## Will I still be able to have children?

Provided you have not had treatment such as ovarian ablation that has left you permanently infertile, you should still be able to have children if you wish. US research suggests that around 10–20 per cent of cases of breast cancer occur in women of childbearing age, and other studies have shown that up to 7 per cent of women who are still fertile after treatment go on to have children.

## If I do get pregnant, will it be safe?

Your long-term outlook if you become pregnant following breast cancer is just as good as it is for women treated for breast cancer who do not become pregnant. For some women getting pregnant after breast cancer provides an added incentive to 'get better'. There's no evidence that pregnancy makes cancer recur or spread more frequently or faster. Nor does there seem to be any increased risk of birth defects or of your child developing cancer, although if your breast cancer was associated with a breast cancer gene there is a risk that your child may have a raised risk of breast, ovarian or colon cancer. In this case you may want to consider genetic counselling to help you weigh up the risks.

Like any couple planning a pregnancy, you and your partner will want to consider all the pros and cons of having a child. This isn't easy at the best of times and it can be doubly difficult when the future is uncertain. You'll also need to think about what your doctors estimate is the risk of your cancer recurring and, difficult though this may be to think about, who will care for your child if you are unlucky and the cancer does come back or spread.

Your breast cancer doctor, surgeon and an obstetrician should all be involved in planning your care during pregnancy and afterwards so as to achieve the best possible outcome for you and your baby.

You may feel you want to give yourself a little time to allow your body the chance to heal and to take steps to get as healthy as you can before trying to conceive. Preconception counselling may help. Your doctor or midwife may be able to refer you, or there are private services.

## Questions to ask your doctor

- What is the risk of my cancer recurring?
- Do you advise me to wait before I try for a pregnancy? Some doctors recommend waiting two or three years to give added confidence that the cancer is not going to return.
- How will having breast cancer affect my antenatal care, the management of birth and delivery and the postnatal period?
- If I'm taking medication, do I need to stop? Doctors recommend that tamoxifen should not be taken during pregnancy. Although there is no proven cause and effect mechanism, some studies have suggested there may be a higher risk of miscarriage, birth defects and stillbirth in women who have taken or are taking tamoxifen.

## Will I be able to breastfeed?

It depends on your treatment. However, many women who have been treated for breast cancer have managed to breastfeed successfully. If you have had a lumpectomy, you will still be able to breastfeed on the side treated, provided an incision was not made around the areola (the area around your nipple) and the ducts leading to the nipple have not been cut. If you have had radiotherapy, you may have problems feeding from the treated breast as the treatment permanently alters the breast tissue. The treated breast won't engorge on the third or fourth day after birth when the milk 'comes in'. This can make your breasts rather lopsided. However, because breastfeeding is a question of supply and demand, you will almost certainly be able to feed on the unaffected side – your baby's suckling will stimulate the breasts to make more milk. If you want to breastfeed, you can get further advice and support from your midwife or a counsellor from one of the breastfeeding organisations such as the NCT or La Leche League.

## What contraception can I use?

Because the female sex hormones oestrogen and progesterone are found in the oral contraceptive Pill and other hormonal methods of contraception, you'll usually be advised to use other forms of contraception. Barrier methods such as condoms and diaphragms are safe and, if used correctly, can be almost as effective as the Pill. IUDs (intrauterine devices) can also be a good choice. Some women who definitely don't want to get pregnant choose sterilisation. Your doctor or family planning clinic can advise you on the different methods that might be suitable.

## What is induced menopause? Is it permanent?

Induced menopause is when oestrogen production by the ovaries is brought to a halt by treatment, rather than by the ovaries running out of eggs as happens at the natural menopause. Most of the hormonal therapies described in the previous chapter induce menopause temporarily. However, when treatment is stopped, oestrogen production resumes and your periods should start again, unless you have undergone the menopause proper during the time you were being treated. Ovarian ablation by surgery or radiotherapy, of course, stops the production of eggs from the ovaries permanently. Some chemotherapy drugs induce premature menopause in some women, although not all. Women aged over 40 who are nearer their natural menopause are more likely to be permanently affected.

## How can I cope with the symptoms of induced menopause?

Many women have found the following helpful:
- Wearing layers and/or using layers on the bed and wearing natural fibres to combat hot flushes.
- Relaxation.
- Exercise.
- Dietary measures – avoiding hot spicy foods, alcohol, caffeinated drinks and large meals for hot flushes.
- Losing weight if you need to may help ease hot flushes.
- Quitting smoking (smokers may have more severe menopausal symptoms).

- Medication – the doctor may be able to prescribe medications for hot flushes, mood swings, vaginal dryness and other menopausal symptoms.
- Vitamins and minerals – some women find taking a multi-vitamin/mineral supplement designed for menopausal women helpful either on its own or with other 'natural' supplements such as red clover. Check with your GP or cancer specialist if you plan to take these in case they interfere with treatment.

**How is my partner likely to be affected by my breast cancer?**

Cancer can overturn the way you and those close to you see yourself and the world. All kinds of factors will affect how your partner reacts: how long you have been together, his or her personality, your response to treatment and the nature of your relationship with each other. It can be hard to watch someone you love struggling with treatment at the same time as wondering if you can deal with the emotional, practical and financial impact of her or his illness. Every person's partner will react differently and his or her reaction may change at different stages in your cancer journey. At first you may both be too overwhelmed by shock to feel anything very much. As time goes on, your partner, like you, may go through a whole range of different emotions: helplessness, guilt, anger, grief, anxiety. Some relationships are severely dented by the strain of coping with cancer. Cancer can sometimes be a convenient peg on which to hang blame for problems that existed beforehand. Having said this, finding a way to talk about problems, and resolving them, can bring couples closer together. If your partner isn't coping well, there is plenty of help out there. CancerBACUP's Cancer Counselling Service can offer one-to-one help and advice, or you may want to seek help from a relationship counselling organisation such as Relate. Breast Cancer Care has an on-line forum for partners wishing to share information and feelings. Alternatively, you may want to consider asking your GP to refer you for counselling or psychotherapy.

**Can positive thinking really help?**

The idea that the way you view the world can affect your risk of developing breast cancer has been batted around ever since the Greek father of medicine, Hippocrates, observed the disease to be a by-product of a melancholic disposition. In more recent times, the idea that stressful events can trigger breast cancer and that approaching the disease with a fighting spirit can improve survival has gained hold. These ideas have proved remarkably tenacious despite the lack of any firm, consistent evidence. The latest research suggests that neither stressful events nor possessing a 'fighting spirit' have any significant bearing on your risk of developing breast cancer or of surviving it. Stressful events, such as bereavement, retirement and so on, are extremely common especially in mid- and later life, the most common time to develop breast cancer, and the idea that feeling upset, frightened, despairing or angry could somehow make your cancer grow can be extremely damaging at a time when people are facing the challenge of dealing with a complex and frightening illness.

According to research carried out at London's Royal Marsden Hospital, the only instance in which mental state appears to affect the outlook is in those who feel their situation is completely hopeless. However, even this finding need not imply straight cause and effect. One possible explanation is that a negative state of mind could influence the immune system in some way. Another is that feelings of helplessness and hopelessness can make it more difficult to seek out the best available treatment or look after yourself. The very last thing you want to be burdened with when facing a disease like breast cancer is the idea that it is somehow 'your fault'. Trying to maintain a positive outlook can be a valuable way of dealing effectively with the challenge of diagnosis and treatment – if that is your coping style. However, you should never feel guilty if you are unable to maintain a positive approach or fear that having a negative attitude has caused your cancer or made it recur.

**Should I let my children see my mastectomy and/or prosthesis?**
A third of women diagnosed with breast cancer in the UK have school-age children and many others have younger or older children. Exactly what you tell your children, when you tell them, how much you tell them and how far you choose to involve them will depend on their age and stage of development, their gender, their individual personalities and your relationship with them. You know your children best, and only you can decide how they are

likely to respond. Younger children who may be around when you are dressing and undressing may be curious and, if you think it would help them to understand what has happened to you better, you may want to offer them the opportunity to see your mastectomy or prosthesis. If you do, you will need to tailor your explanation to their age and level of understanding. However, be aware that not all children – even adolescent or adult ones – will want to see. Adolescent children who are struggling to come to terms with their own emerging sexuality may feel embarrassed or afraid. Older daughters in particular may be afraid of the implications of your diagnosis and what it means to their own risk of developing breast cancer. Denial – pretending something is not happening – is one way to cope. It doesn't mean they don't care.

- Allow your children to share the experience of breast cancer to the extent that they are able and that is helpful to you.
- Take into account your children's individual differences and tailor your approach to their needs.
- Give your children time and space to come to terms with your illness in their own way.
- Try not to feel hurt or rejected if a child refuses to look at your mastectomy or prosthesis.
- Breast Cancer Care has information on talking to children and what children at different ages understand (see p.259).

**I don't seem to be recovering well emotionally: is counselling available?**

The experience of having breast cancer evokes a whole range of emotions from the time of diagnosis onwards. Anxiety, fear, irritability, sadness and despair are common and can at times feel overwhelming. A diagnosis of breast cancer raises a whole host of questions: How will I cope with treatment? Will the cancer return or spread? Am I going to die? What impact will cancer have on the rest of my life, my job, my finances, my relationships with partner and/or children and with family and friends? How you cope with your emotional needs will depend on what works best for you. You may prefer to deal with your emotions privately or with the help of family and friends. However, if you feel you need additional help, there are many different options. These include:

- **Individual counselling/psychotherapy**. It can be helpful to talk to someone outside your family and friends who is trained to listen without judging you, and who may be able to suggest strategies for dealing with your emotions. Most breast cancer nurses are trained in basic counselling techniques. For more specific help you may want to be referred to a specialist counsellor or therapist with a special interest in cancer. The breast care nurse, your GP or one of the breast cancer organisations such as Breast Cancer Care should be able to point you in the right direction.
- **Support groups**. Some breast care nurses run support groups within the hospital. Breast Cancer Care can also tell you if there are any support groups in your area. Support groups can be a useful forum in which to share ideas with other women in the same situation. There are different types and you may want to try one or more to find which best suits you.
- **One-to-one support**. Your breast care nurse or organisations such as Breast Cancer Care can put you in touch with women in your area who have or have had breast cancer. Keeping a journal or finding support from family, friends and support groups may also be helpful.

# Follow-up care and recurrence

After your immediate treatment has ended, you will still be invited to your breast cancer unit for check-ups every so often to see how you are recovering and to check that there has been no recurrence of the cancer. A typical schedule of appointments would be a six-monthly check-up for five years and then annually after that. These check-ups will include:

- **Taking a history:** The doctor will ask how you are feeling. Tell him or her about any changes in the treated area or the other breast and any unusual symptoms.
- **Physical examination.**
- **Mammography and breast ultrasound** will be carried out at regular intervals. A typical pattern might be to have a mammogram annually for the first five years and then every two years after that.

It is not usual to have other screening tests such as CT and other types of scans or blood tests as a routine unless there are grounds for suspecting there may be a recurrence.

**What will happen when I have been cancer free for five years?**
In some centres you will have yearly check-ups for the rest of your life, in some you will be discharged, while in others you will be discharged after ten years. However, after five years the risk of recurrence becomes less and less.

**Questions to ask your doctor**

- How often do you recommend I attend for check-ups? What will these involve?
- How can I tell if aches and pains are normal or symptoms of recurrence?
- Will I have any specialist tests if I don't have any symptoms?
- If I think cancer has returned, what tests might you do?
- How accurate are these?
- How long will I have to wait for testing?
- How soon will I have the results?

**How can I check myself after a mastectomy or lumpectomy?**

It is virtually impossible for a surgeon to remove every piece of breast tissue, so even if you have had a mastectomy it is important to continue to be breast aware so you can pick up any potentially suspicious changes. The technique is similar to that used for ordinary breast examination.

- Lie down and raise your arm and using the opposite hand feel the scar using three or four fingers and pressing gently with a circular motion (just as you do when examining the non-affected breast) along the length of the scar and the tissue around it. In the case of breast reconstruction, feel carefully along the scar around the edges of an implant or a flap.

- Work your way over the whole area, under the collarbone and under your arm.

- You are looking for any thickening, masses, swollen lymph nodes or unusual lumps under the skin, nipple discharge (particularly if it is bloody), and especially any change from a previous examination.

- Note any new lumps, bumps, hard areas or thickenings and any unusual pain or tenderness.

- Now stand up and check the area in the mirror. Be on the look-out for skin changes such as dimpling, puckering or retraction of the skin, a change in skin colour and/or texture.

- If you have had a lumpectomy and still have a nipple, check it, noting any discharge (especially if it is bloody), retraction of the nipple or scaly skin on or around it.

- It is quite normal for scar tissue to feel rather lumpy and hard and for the skin around it to pucker slightly. Get to know what is normal for you so you can note anything unusual, or any changes from your previous self-examination, and report it to your doctor.

**What is recurrent breast cancer?**

Recurrent breast cancer is cancer that returns after the original, or primary, breast cancer has been treated. It may affect the treated breast, the chest wall or another part of the body.

### How likely is breast cancer to recur?

Your exact risk of recurrence will be related to several factors, including whether your original cancer was in situ or invasive, the size of the tumour, how far advanced it was, and the presence and number of lymph nodes that were involved. Most women with a small tumour with no lymph node involvement have no recurrence 10 years or more after treatment. If your initial breast cancer was a fast-growing, aggressive type with several lymph nodes involved, or if you had inflammatory breast cancer, you are more likely to experience a recurrence within a shorter time.

Sometimes a new breast cancer can occur several years after the original cancer. This may be in a different area of the breast or of a different type to the original cancer. Second cancers are regarded as new cancers, although how they are treated may depend on how the first cancer was treated, as certain treatments such as radiotherapy cannot be repeated in the same areas, and drugs such as anthracycline chemotherapy cannot be used again.

### What is the risk of another tumour developing in the same or my other breast?

Recurrence in the same breast may be due to cells left after surgery or a new tumour that has developed. This is known as local recurrence. Radiotherapy reduces the risk of this happening. Sometimes a new cancer develops in another part of the treated breast or in the untreated breast.

### When might breast cancer recur?

Most recurrences happen within the first two to five years after initial treatment. However, cancer can return at any time – sometimes as many as 20 or 30 years later. This is why, although you may want to forget about having had breast cancer and get on with your life, it is important to take advantage of any follow-up care recommended.

### If the cancer does come back, what part of my body might it affect?

Breast cancer can recur in virtually any part of the body. Recurrence falls into three different categories:

**Local recurrence:** Most often breast cancer recurs in the same area as the original tumour. Most doctors do not consider local recurrence a spread of breast cancer but rather to be an extension of the first cancer caused by a few cells being left behind after treatment.

**Regional recurrence:** Less often, cancer recurs in the area around the breast, usually in the lymph glands situated in the armpit, under the breastbone, or above the collarbone, or it can recur in the chest wall. Doctors usually consider this to be more serious than local recurrence as it is a sign that cancer cells have passed into the lymphatic system and could spread further.

**Secondary breast cancer/metastatic spread/distant spread:** Breast cancer may also recur in other parts of the body – most often affecting the bones, the liver, the lungs or occasionally the brain. The cells don't usually spread to all these places at once, although it is possible to have secondary breast cancer in more than one site.

### How might a local recurrence be treated?

**Following a lumpectomy:** You will usually be recommended to have a mastectomy, possibly followed by chemotherapy. Endocrine therapy may be restarted or altered depending on individual circumstances. Radiotherapy is sometimes given, but only if it wasn't used after the lumpectomy as it cannot generally be delivered twice to the same treatment field.

**Following a mastectomy:** If the lump can be removed, then an operation is usually performed and the recurrent cancer removed. If removal is not possible, the scar line or chest wall may be treated with radiotherapy (see above) and/or chemotherapy or other systemic (whole body) therapies. Sometimes after chemotherapy or radiotherapy the recurrence shrinks and an operation to remove all the tissue is then performed.

### What are the symptoms of regional recurrence and how may it be treated?

Most often a regional recurrence is found in an axillary (underarm) lymph node that was not removed during your original treatment. Treatment may involve simply removing the cancerous node. Regional recurrences may also occur elsewhere in the region around the breast such as the muscles of the chest wall, the lymph nodes under the breastbone, between the ribs, above the collarbone and surrounding the neck. These are usually treated with a combination of radiotherapy (if not already given) and chemotherapy or hormonal treatment.

### Can secondary/metastatic breast cancer be cured?

Unfortunately, once cancer has spread beyond the lymph glands it can never be entirely eliminated, although it can be controlled and effectively treated and may go into remission completely, i.e. no evidence of it is present (although it will eventually return). Often people live for many years with metastatic disease. Breast cancer cells that have spread to other parts of the body are still breast cancer cells – even if they are in the lungs or the bones. This can be confusing, but it is important to know because it affects the treatment you will receive. The treatment for secondary breast cancer that has spread to the bone is quite different from the treatment for primary bone cancer (cancer arising in the bone cells).

### How do breast cancer cells spread to other parts of the body?

Breast cancer cells travel around the body in two ways:

- In the bloodstream.
- Via the lymphatic system.

Once the cells have spread elsewhere, they may begin to form a secondary tumour. This doesn't always happen straightaway. Sometimes the cells can lie dormant, often for many years, before beginning to form a tumour. What triggers metastasised cells to reactivate is still a mystery, and the subject of much research.

### What are the signs and symptoms of secondary breast cancer?

Secondary breast cancer is not a single condition, and the precise symptoms will depend on which organs are affected. It is natural when you have had a serious disease like cancer to want to know which symptoms might indicate recurrence or spread and which are simply the normal aches and pains that everybody gets. Don't be afraid to bother your doctor if you are worried. Often symptoms are due to something completely unrelated to the breast cancer. It is better to find that it was a false alarm than to ignore something that may potentially be serious.

# Lucy Edwards

When I saw my consultant for the first time, I was still reeling from the shock and distress of discovering I had breast cancer. I was 30, and had learnt just a few minutes before that what I'd thought was a cyst had turned out to be cancer. I had been sent to the One Stop Clinic in Norwich where you can be examined and diagnosed the same day, so the news had come very quickly indeed. The consultant was very cool and pragmatic, but I was crying. The hospital breast care nurse sat with me and supported me, while he was very cool and dispassionate.

While the consultant explained my choices to me, he also wrote them down, which I was later to be grateful for. I was so numb with shock it was hard to take in what he was saying. When I left, the consultant shook my hand and said a few encouraging words, but it took me a long time to build up a relationship with him. I now trust his medical judgement completely but do feel that his 'bedside manner' could be better.

I knew I wanted a family, so I chose a form of chemotherapy that would not affect my fertility. However, my consultant hadn't suggested that I have some ovarian tissue frozen privately to enable me to have children in the future and I was angry at having to find this out for myself. He said he wasn't aware of the scheme. But when I told him I wanted to do this he was supportive and we scheduled my treatment around it.

At first, my tumour responded well, but when later the cancer returned I had to have a mastectomy. The surgeon who did this was a lot warmer – he could actually make jokes and make me smile. It really does help a lot when someone does that.

After this operation, I was ready to ask my consultant 'the hard questions'. I asked if he thought it would come back and he said yes. We decided to leave more chemotherapy in reserve. I found this very strange – from having so much treatment I was now having none. It felt a bit like flying without a safety net.

Two years later my progress has been good. Rather than seeing my consultant monthly, I now see him every nine months. If I have another lump, he is confident I am body aware and would spot it quickly. He also advised against regular blood tests, as they are not always accurate and can cause distress. I also have some criticisms of my consultant's approach, mainly to do with his tone and manner. When talking about life or death situations, the consultant sounded almost blithe about it; maybe he's just more honest about death than I was used to. He said I should not try for a baby for five years. I asked, why five? He used the words 'to ensure the survival of the mother', which I found a bit chilling. Consultants can forget you are not a medical professional and cannot understand their arguments quickly. They can also sound very cold but I can understand why. I feel it is not his job to become emotionally involved, though it can be very frustrating for the patient. The relationship between us is now warmer because it has been built up over time.

## What investigations might be done?

A variety of different tests can be performed to check whether the cancer has spread. The precise ones will vary depending on where the cancer is suspected to have spread to. They include:

### Blood tests

A variety can be done to measure how different organs are functioning. These may include a liver function test and a test to detect calcium in the blood caused by calcium leaching from the bones in metastatic breast cancer in the bone.

### X-rays

Different kinds may be performed. For example, a chest X-ray may be done to show whether cancer has spread to the lungs. A bone X-ray may be done, although it may not be sensitive enough to detect small tumours.

### CT (CAT) scan

A type of X-ray which builds up a 3-D picture of various body organs or structures. It is used to identify the site of a tumour and check for spread. It can be used to check for secondary cancer in the brain, liver and other organs.

### Bone scan

This is more sensitive than X-ray at identifying secondary cancers in small areas of bone. A small quantity of a mild radioactive agent is injected into a vein and travels around your body via the bloodstream. More radioactivity is absorbed by areas of bone affected by cancer and this will show up on the scan.

### Magnetic resonance imaging (MRI)

Magnetism is used to build up a cross-section of different parts of the body. You will have to lie extremely still on a couch which is slid into a long drum-like chamber. This can take as long as an hour and can be rather claustrophobic, so tell the radiographer if you dislike enclosed spaces. As the scanning process is noisy, you'll be given earplugs.

### Liver scan

A type of ultrasound scan.

## What are tumour marker tests and will I have any?

'Tumour markers' are produced by the tumour or the body in response to the cancer and can often be detected in higher than normal amounts in the bloodstream if a tumour is present.

Measuring tumour markers can sometimes help the doctor in diagnosing recurrence, although there can be other reasons why tumour marker levels are raised so it won't be used alone. It can also help the doctor decide how the tumour is responding to treatment, allowing him or her to plan the most appropriate treatment. It is still fairly early days for tumour markers in breast cancer, although in some other cancers such as prostate cancer in men or ovarian cancer in women, they are of more use in treatment decisions.

## What factors will my doctor take into account when recommending treatment?

The doctor will take the following into account:

**Factors affecting you**

These include how old you are, your overall state of health and whether you have any other medical conditions that might affect your health or treatment. Whether or not you have been through the menopause is likely to be another factor, as pre-menopausally you are likely to have high levels of female hormones circulating in your bloodstream and this means that different hormonal treatments are used in pre- and post-menopausal women with secondary breast cancer.

**Factors to do with the secondary cancer**

These include:

**Nature of the secondary cancer:** The doctor will assess the secondary cancer and whether it is slow- or fast-growing, together with what other treatment you had originally.

**Site of the spread:** Cancers in certain parts of the body respond best to different kinds of treatment. For instance, secondary breast cancer in the bones, lymph nodes, skin and fatty tissue is often treated with hormonal therapies, whereas chemotherapy is used more often for cancer that has spread to the liver or lungs. Radiotherapy is often used to treat cancer that has affected specific bones, parts of the brain or skin close to the breast or mastectomy scar (provided it has not already been given). Radiotherapy is most effective as a local treatment for localised areas of recurrent cancer.

**Cell type (histology):** The nature of the cancer cells, for example their hormonal status and whether they are oestrogen receptor positive, determines whether a cancer will be sensitive to hormonal therapy.

## Questions to ask your doctor

- What are my treatment options?
- How do the various treatments work?
- What is the goal of treatment? Is it aimed at curing my cancer, helping me live longer or dealing with symptoms?
- What can I expect treatment to achieve?
- What side-effects can I expect from treatment?
- Are these likely to be temporary or permanent?
- Will I have to be admitted to hospital for treatment?
- If treatments can be given in outpatients, how long are they likely to take?
- How many treatments am I likely to need?
- Will I be able to get to the hospital under my own steam or will somebody need to take me?
- How is treatment likely to affect other aspects of my life such as my diet, my work and my sex life?
- How soon do I have to decide on treatment?
- Can I have a second opinion?
- Is there anything I can do to help myself?

### How involved can I be in treatment decisions?

Being involved in treatment decisions can help you feel more in control. You may want to discuss the various options with the breast care nurse and with those close to you and/or to do your own research in books or on the Internet. If you don't want to be involved in treatment decisions, however, this is perfectly OK. Coming to terms with secondary breast cancer is often extremely difficult after the hope that your cancer had been conquered. Having to make decisions about treatment can be an extra burden you may feel you don't want to carry. Try to keep your doctor informed about how you are feeling and don't feel a failure if you change your mind.

### How am I likely to feel if secondary cancer is diagnosed?

A diagnosis of secondary breast cancer can be an especially bitter blow and it may take time to come to terms with it. It is natural to feel angry and depressed. Bear in mind that although secondary breast cancer is not normally curable it can be controlled, often for many years. If you are having trouble coping with your feelings, the breast care nurse may be able to refer you to a counsellor or a member of the palliative care team who is experienced in talking to people with secondary cancer.

## How effective are the treatments for secondary breast cancer?

Treatments for secondary breast cancer can be extremely effective. However, it is important to recognise that there is usually no cure. Currently there are many women living full, active lives with secondary breast cancer and, as treatments improve still further, there are likely to be many more.

## What if treatment stops working?

One of the features of secondary tumours is that they can eventually become resistant to treatment. Fortunately, secondary breast cancer often responds to more than one treatment, so if one stops working there is always another that can be tried. Your doctor is likely to choose the simplest treatment with the fewest side-effects first and then move on to others if this stops being effective. However, sooner or later the doctor may advise you that no more active treatment is possible, or you may decide you would prefer to discontinue treatment. In this case there are plenty of ways you can be helped. You'll find lots of advice in the next chapter.

## Will I be in pain?

Advanced breast cancer does not always cause pain and much will depend on where in the body you develop secondaries. Pain may be especially troublesome if you have secondary breast cancer in a bone. If you are in pain, do seek the help of your doctor. There is a whole range of painkilling drugs and other measures that may be taken to help keep pain to a minimum and possibly banish it altogether.

## How might pain be controlled?

There are a number of painkilling drugs. In addition there is a range of non-drug treatments. These include:

- Radiotherapy.
- Transcutaneous nerve stimulation (TENS).
- Nerve blocks using drugs injected into the central nervous system such as epidural.

- Complementary therapies such as acupuncture, hypnotherapy, visualisation and other techniques designed to help you relax.

Your GP or consultant can refer you to a specialist pain clinic or a consultant who is experienced in symptom control. If you are prescribed painkillers, bear in mind that it may take a certain amount of trial and error to find the exact medication to control your pain most effectively, so be patient, and if something doesn't work, tell the doctor.

- Painkillers are usually most effective when they are taken regularly, even if pain has been eased, as their effects build up in the body.

- All drugs have side-effects as well as benefits. These are usually mild and may ease over time. However, if side-effects become troublesome, consult the doctor: there may be another drug that could be prescribed or self-help measures that will minimise them.

- If a painkiller isn't effective in alleviating pain, tell the doctor. There are many different types and they will usually be able to prescribe a different one or ones if your current painkillers are not effective, or don't suit you for any reason.

- Pain is always worse when you are tense. Techniques such as relaxation, guided visualisation and massage, and simple self-help techniques like self-massage and taking a warm bath can help relax you and thereby ease pain.

# Palliative care

If you are told that no further medical treatment is possible to control your cancer, it does not mean nothing further can be done to help you. Palliative care is given to alleviate symptoms or problems arising from cancer when it can no longer be actively treated. Unlike active treatment that aims to bring about a long-term remission or slow the progress of cancer, palliative care is not expected to eliminate the disease but to enable you – and those who care for you – to live life as fully as possible, despite any limitations imposed by your cancer. The particular treatments and the type of support you will receive will depend on where you live and your individual needs. However, medical treatments are often less aggressive and gentler than those used in active treatment because the emphasis is on the quality of life rather than on cure.

Aspects of palliative care include:

- controlling pain and other distressing symptoms of advanced cancer
- using a range of strategies, from medical treatments to complementary therapies, to help alleviate physical and emotional problems
- supporting you and your family practically and emotionally

**When will I have palliative care and will I automatically be offered it?**

In the past palliative care was provided only after all efforts to halt cancer had failed. Today, improvements in medical care and treatments mean that it is possible to live for many years with breast cancer. Ideally, palliative care should now be an integral part of the care offered to everyone with advanced cancer, not just those approaching the end of life.

**How widely available is palliative care?**

Shortages of funding mean that many services are stretched, and it can be hard to find out exactly what is available and how to access it. The Government is committed to extending palliative care by training more district nurses to help them support people with cancer at home, and improving access to palliative care in inner cities and rural areas. Eight palliative care partnership projects have been set up to spread knowledge and encourage good practice, and the National Council for Hospices and Specialist Palliative Care has been funded to help cancer networks work with voluntary hospices to assess local needs and develop plans to meet them.

Until these initiatives are in place, it may take a certain amount of determination and assertiveness to obtain the services you are entitled to. Your local social services department should be able to tell you what's on offer in your area and advise you on how to get different kinds of non-medical help.

## What can I expect from palliative care?

Palliative care teams may be based at the local hospital or hospice. The members of this team can help you and those who care for you in several ways. For example, they may:

- Explain what medical and other techniques can help alleviate pain.
- Provide advice on different treatments for symptoms and advice on dealing with potential side-effects.
- Provide you and your carers with emotional support.
- Spend time with your carers and enable them to care for and support you most effectively.
- Provide advice and information on practicalities such as financial issues and benefits.
- Help allay fear by providing information about your illness and what to expect at the end of life.
- Encourage you to be open and to share your feelings with those close to you at your own pace and in your own time.

## What support services may be on offer?

Support services come from three main sources:

- The NHS, for example your GP, district nurse, hospital or hospice support care team.
- Your local social services department (or social work department if you live in Scotland) for example social worker/care manager.

- Voluntary organisations, for example Macmillan, Marie Curie and Sue Ryder who all have specialist nurses working in hospitals, hospices and the community.

Exactly how much support you receive and how it will be delivered will depend on where you live and how support services are organised in your area. However, if you need extra care or help, you will usually be able to access it through one of these routes.

### If I need looking after at home, what kind of support will be available to those caring for me?

Again, this will depend on where you live and what kind of help and support you need.

- **Your GP.** Once you are based at home, your GP will be in overall charge of your medical care. They will be able to prescribe any drugs you need, organise for nursing care and arrange for you to go into a hospital or hospice if this is necessary.
- **Nursing care.** Your doctor or the hospital can arrange for a district nurse to visit and administer any regular drugs or injections, change dressings and provide nursing care. Where necessary, they can instruct your carer in simple basic tasks such as washing, lifting and personal care and can also organise for any special aids, equipment or extra services, such as a continence adviser or physiotherapist. Your GP, hospital or hospice may also be able to organise for a Marie Curie or Macmillan nurse, who is specially trained in caring for people with cancer, to visit. They can spend the night or some of the day with you, giving your carer the chance to catch up on sleep or take a break. Macmillan nurses specialise in pain and symptom control and can also provide you and/or your carer(s) with counselling and emotional support. If needed, for example if your carer has to go out to work, and if funds run to it, private nursing care may be available through a local nursing agency. Your carer can get details of recommended agencies from the local social services department or a carers' or cancer support group.
- **Non-medical services.** The social worker or care manager can help set the wheels in motion for a variety of non-medical support services such as meals on wheels, home help, personal care and laundry. They can organise for an occupational

# Gill Oliver, Macmillan Cancer Relief

In order to understand the current role of Macmillan Cancer Relief in the field of palliative care it important to consider the historical context. Some twenty or thirty years ago the expression 'terminal care' was common place – care at the end of life. It was at this point in a cancer diagnosis that the special skills of the Macmillan Nurse were put to good effect, although the link with death and dying was sometimes a cause for anxiety amongst patients and relatives.

An alternative word was needed and the term palliative care (from the Latin word 'to cloak') came in to being. Palliative care is an inclusive term covering a range of patient needs – physical, emotional, psychological and social. Palliative Care also includes the assessment and management of symptoms associated with a diagnosis of cancer. Although initially palliative care carried with it a similar stigma to 'terminal care' latterly it is seen as an essential part of care and support from the point of diagnosis onwards.

As we move to the 21st century we are looking for even more accurate ways of describing the care that patients and their families need, and we are beginning to talk about Supportive and Palliative care. This description places the person affected by cancer as the central focus at all times. The concept of Supportive and Palliative care is not specific to a particular type of cancer or even a particular disease. The aim is always to ensure that efficient and effective care and support is provided, and that people affected by cancer are helped and supported to go on with their lives whether their cancer treatment is still continuing or has been completed. The emphasis is on 'living' with cancer and their needs may be more to do with practical issues such as help with transport, childcare or managing the house and garden rather than clinical care for their disease. The precise definitions of Supportive and Palliative care have yet to be agreed. The National

Council for Hospice and Specialist Care Services is currently concluding a piece of work to provide precise definitions of these two terms. However, the words we use to describe services are of less importance than the work required to ensure that an individual affected by cancer is able to have access to the range of support and care services that he or she needs to live more easily with the effects of a cancer diagnosis and its treatment.

The principles underpinning Macmillan Cancer Relief's activity in the field of cancer and palliative care are those of collaboration and partnership. We are a development organisation, working with others to add value, to influence the planning and implementation of a variety of services and to identify gaps where new services really can make a change for the better. The wealth of experience, skill and knowledge that Macmillan people have built up over the 90 years of the organisation's existence is brought to bear on strategic planning and policy formation, and in influencing the establishment of a range of innovative projects and services from new buildings to Carers' Schemes and posts for doctors and nurses, and from Information Centres to Patient Partnership Groups.

Through working in partnership with others, through adding value and through building on the expertise and experience of its staff and postholders, Macmillan Cancer Relief looks forward to a time when everyone affected by cancer has access to the very best cancer treatment care and support.

therapist to call, who can advise on and help organise any special equipment such as wheelchairs or adaptations to your home that can help make everyday life easier. The social worker should also be able to help with practicalities such as advice on benefits, holidays and respite care. Many social workers have counselling skills and help support you and your carer(s) emotionally.

### How will I cope if I live alone?

It can be particularly hard to cope with advanced breast cancer if you live alone and you will almost certainly have days when you feel alone and depressed. It can be hard to ask for help if you have always been used to being independent. Friends and relatives will often be willing to help if they can, and you should not feel afraid to let them know the ways in which they can be most useful. You should be eligible for some or all of the supportive services already mentioned. CancerBACUP and Breast Cancer Care can give you further advice.

### Is there anything I can do to help myself?

Even while you are receiving medical care, advances in pain control mean you will often be able to stay independent and you may well be able to continue many of the things you enjoy doing such as work, sport or hobbies, travel and spending time with your friends and/or family. However, as your cancer progresses, there may come a time when you have to lean more on those around you. This can be difficult if you have always prided yourself on your independence. Bear in mind that whatever happens you are still a unique individual with desires, wishes and rights. Even if you are confined to bed there are ways in which you can continue to exert control over your life. Making decisions about your care, your activities, what you want to eat and what you need for your comfort and communicating your needs to those around you can help you feel much more in charge of your life, whatever the stage of your cancer.

### Will I be entitled to any benefits?

Cancer, like any other illness that continues for a long time, can put considerable pressure on your finances. As well as coping with loss of income incurred by you and possibly your partner, you may well have to find the cash for extra expenses such as heating, laundry services, travel to and from hospital and so on. Fortunately, you and/or your carer may be eligible for a number of different benefits.

- **Government benefits.** You may be eligible for Income Support, Incapacity Benefit, Disabled Living Allowance or Invalid Care Allowance, which can be paid to your partner, and/or a number of other benefits. If you are on Income Support, you may be able to claim a Community Care Grant for costs like travel, bedding and a washing machine or dryer. You can get specific advice and information from the Benefits Agency (address in phone book), Citizens Advice Bureaux, social worker/care manager or other local agencies such as welfare rights unit, law centre or cancer support group. The DSS Helpline on 0800 666 555 should also be able to give you specific advice.
- **Macmillan Cancer Relief grants.** The charity Macmillan Cancer Relief awards grants to help meet the costs of home care, sitters, home nursing, travel expenses, holidays, heating, clothing, bedding, telephone installation and bills to single people with less than £6,000 in savings or couples whose savings are less than £8,000. The charity also offers smaller sums for items such as a fan heater or a liquidiser. Your Macmillan nurse, social worker or district nurse can help you apply.
- **Other charities.** Several charities provide financial help for people in need. The book *A Guide to Grants for Individuals in Need* gives details.

### I'm being referred to a hospice. Does that mean I am going to die soon?

A hospice is a place where the doctors, nurses and other staff are specially trained in palliative care. Although hospices were originally set up to help people facing death, today they have a much broader remit. You may be referred to a hospice for a short stay when you need extra help with symptom control, for example, or if your carer(s) need a break. Some hospitals have special palliative care units offering similar services to a hospice. Some hospices have Day Centres which you can go to for a couple of days a week, and many have Home Care Teams, consisting of doctors and nurses from the hospice who will come to your home.

The advantage of spending time in a hospice is that it is a place that is dedicated to providing symptom control, and the staff are experienced in the special concerns and issues facing people with advanced cancer and their families, and have more time than the staff on a busy cancer unit usually have to listen to you and cater for your needs. And, contrary to what you might imagine, hospices are not gloomy places. Most hospices are calm, pleasant places with attractive grounds. Many are purpose-built with kitchens, sitting rooms and somewhere relatives can stay.

**How can I find out more about my local hospice and will I have to pay to go there?**
Your GP, district or cancer care nurse or the Hospice Information Service should be able to give you details of your local hospice. Care is free.

**Will I have to wait to go into a hospice?**
Occasionally you may have to be put on a waiting list. However, you won't usually have to wait longer than a couple of weeks or so.

# Your rights

In the past, variations in prescribing practices and shortages of specialists meant the chances of getting effective treatment and the latest drugs often depended on where you lived. In the last few years the Government has made strenuous efforts to put an end to 'postcode prescribing' and variations in care through the development of its National Cancer Plan, which sets out exactly how people with various types of cancers should be cared for. Several developments mean that you can now be assured that the treatments and drugs you receive at your hospital are just as good as those you would receive anywhere else:

- **Cancer Networks.** In England, cancer care is organised into 34 Cancer Networks, with one or two key hospitals in each area which can provide all types of cancer care and treatment, including specialised treatments such as radiotherapy. Other hospitals in the area provide standard tests and treatments. If more specialised tests or treatment are needed, you will usually be referred to the major hospital or hospitals. The system is similar in Scotland and Wales, which each have three Networks providing co-ordinated care. Northern Ireland is currently integrating its six Trusts into one Cancer Network.

- **Higher standards of treatment.** The Government's first ever *Manual of Cancer Services Standards*, which sets out standards for treatment, should eventually iron out differences in standards of cancer care. The services provided by each NHS hospital have been reviewed by teams of experts and action plans set up to ensure that they meet the standards set, as well as mechanisms for tracking quality and efficacy of treatments.

- **NICE (National Institute for Clinical Excellence).** This is the body which since 1999 has had the task of monitoring all the evidence on existing drugs used to treat diseases such as breast cancer and assessing the value of new ones, to ensure that doctors have reliable, up-to-date guidance on the latest proven treatments. The aim is to make sure that no matter where you live you get the best possible treatment. The system isn't perfect and there have been what some consider unacceptable delays in assessing certain treatments. What's more, because NICE includes cost-effectiveness among its criteria for assessing new treatments, this can affect its recommendations. You can check the NICE website to see that your unit or health authority is following guidelines and what treatments have been approved: www.nice.org.uk

- **More doctors and nurses.** There are plans under the National Cancer Plan to train more specialist doctors and other staff so that you can be seen quickly and have enough time to discuss your illness. The Government has set a target of nearly 1,000 extra cancer consultants by 2006 and initiatives are under way to train staff in skills and areas traditionally carried out by other specialists, such as radiotherapy, breast screening and cell analysis.

### How do British drugs and treatments measure up to those available in the United States or Europe?

The main proven drugs and treatments for breast cancer used in the UK are essentially the same as those used in the US and Europe, although there may be slight differences in the way they are prescribed and when different treatments are given. However, there are many experimental drugs in the pipeline and these may differ from country to country. Some drugs might also be available elsewhere before they become available here – herceptin is an example, which has been available in France for some time. If you've read about one of these in the newspapers, you may be wondering why you haven't been prescribed it. The first thing to bear in mind is that only a tiny proportion of drugs tested ever produce a viable new treatment. And even those that do tend only to offer a small gain on tried and tested therapies. Journalists often hail treatments as breakthroughs before all the advantages and disadvantages are fully known. It takes many years to test a new drug or treatment and there are few that are truly revolutionary – whatever you might have read in the paper. Usually there will be good reasons why you have been recommended a particular drug or treatment and, if you are unsure why a particular treatment has been prescribed, it is a good idea to discuss it with your doctor before assuming that it's not as good as something you could get elsewhere.

Having said all this, in the past few years there has been genuine cause for excitement, with new knowledge about the human genome (the gene sequence that makes up human beings) and how these affect the chain of events that leads to cancer, resulting in the development of potential new treatments. The first of a new generation of 'molecular' drugs, such as herceptin, that work in a different way to conventional chemotherapy are beginning to come onto the market. In years to come the number of such drugs will increase, making it possible to tailor treatments more closely to individuals using their unique genetic profile. With the development of such treatments, cancer is gradually being transformed from a disease that carried a death sentence to a chronic condition such as diabetes that can be managed.

## Should I consider going abroad for treatment?

Many European countries have a surfeit of doctors, there are more hospital beds, less time from initial consultation to seeing a specialist and no waiting lists for treatment. According to a new law, UK citizens do have the right to seek treatment in the European Union on the NHS, if there is an excessive wait here or if there is good reason why you should have a particular 'well-established' treatment not available here. Sadly, this rules out most of the new drugs or treatments you might have read about.

Seeking treatment abroad can appear an attractive proposition, especially if the NHS might foot the bill. However, there are several factors to bear in mind before you go ahead.

- The NHS will only pay for treatments backed by evidence that they are of proven value – not for trials or experimental therapies.
- It can take time to organise all the formalities, so you will need to consider whether you would be better off waiting for treatment here.
- You also need to consider the potential stress of travelling and being treated far from home, family and friends.

If you do decide to go ahead, there are several steps you need to take:

- Establish where you wish to go and who you want to perform the treatment. You can get information from other people who have been treated abroad, from your NHS consultant or the Department of Health website (Health Advice for Travellers).

- Speak to your consultant. They must agree that the treatment is necessary and that you cannot get it in this country. This means that you must speak to your breast surgeon if you are contemplating surgery and the clinical or medical oncologist if you are contemplating chemotherapy.
- The consultant must then provide your local Health Authority with evidence both that the treatment is necessary and that it cannot be given in this country.

**Within the EU**

- To obtain treatment in the EU you will need to get hold of an E112 certificate from the Department of Health. To do this, contact your local Health Authority's finance or contracts department, who will contact the Department of Health on your behalf.
- While you are waiting for clearance, you should contact the hospital and consultant you wish to treat you.

**For treatment in the US or outside the EU**

- You will need to get the approval of your local Health Authority, and they will need to apply to the International Branch of the Department of Health. Again, the treatment has to be 'well established' to merit consideration.

You could of course decide to pay for treatment abroad, but this would almost certainly be extremely expensive, as it would include the cost of treatment plus travelling and accommodation in the country you have chosen. If you have the funds, you may decide it is worth it. However, as before, bear in mind that your cancer care team will have planned your care extremely carefully to ensure you get the best treatment for you, and going abroad won't necessarily mean that you get better treatment.

**Pros and cons of treatment abroad**

**Pros**

- Faster treatment.
- Existence of treatments that may not yet be available in the UK (although the NHS won't pay for these if they are experimental).

**Cons**

- Difficulty of finding hospital/specialist and lack of knowledge of facilities and competence.
- NHS won't pay for treatments not of proven value so you won't be able to participate in trials.

- You have to pay for travel even if the NHS pays for treatment.
- Being away from family and friends at a time when you may need extra support.
- Possible language difficulties if complications occur.
- Problems if a complication occurs after you have returned home.
- Stress of travelling, which can be uncomfortable if you've had surgery and may predispose you to complications such as deep vein thrombosis.
- Long-term follow-up more difficult.

## Can I find out what research is being carried out?

Your doctor may know some of the research being carried out. Alternatively, if you have access to the Internet, you might like to check some of the specialist sites. In 2002 the two giants of cancer research in the UK – the Cancer Research Fund and the Imperial Cancer Research Fund Breast Cancer UK – merged to form Cancer Research UK. You can find details on:
www.cancerhelp.org.uk/trials/trials/default.asp

The National Cancer Institute register of trials lists all the clinical trials in progress in this country. Check the website at:
www.ctu.mrc.ac.uk/ukcccr/

The US National Cancer Institute has the largest register of clinical trials, including some that are being carried out in the UK. The website is: www.cancer.gov/clinical_trials/

Another useful US site is: www.controlled-trials.com/. This is an international database of randomised controlled trials in all aspects of healthcare, including cancer.

## What about a cure?

Many cancer doctors are somewhat wary of the word 'cure', because even when breast cancer seems to have gone away it has a habit of coming back again, even many years later. For this reason, many prefer the term 'remission' to 'cure'. Having said this, most recurrences tend to occur within the first couple of years after diagnosis and doctors will often describe you as 'cured' if you have been cancer free for five, or sometimes 10, years.

## Is there likely to be a cure for breast cancer in the future?

Breast cancer is an extremely complex disease, so it is unlikely that there will be a cure in the near future. However, a great deal has been learnt about the disease in the past few years and with the research that is going on currently there's certainly a real prospect of keeping cancer at bay, transforming it into a chronic disease that can be controlled and that people can live with, often for many years. With treatments such as tamoxifen and the new biological treatments such as herceptin, this is already happening to a large extent, and more of these drugs are in development and should be available in the not too distant future.

## How do I complain if I think I've been poorly treated?

If you are unhappy with the care you have received in hospital or from any of your doctors, you have a right to complain. In the first instance you may want to complain informally to the person concerned, or if you don't feel able to talk to them, with a member of staff such as the breast care nurse. If you feel this would not help, you can contact your local Patient Advisory and Liaison Service (PALS). These are the local watchdog bodies which have been set up to replace Community Health Councils (during 2002). You should be able to get details from the hospital, your GP's surgery or Directory Enquiries. A friend or relative can also contact PALS on your behalf, although they must have your written permission to discuss your case. A representative of PALS can visit you in hospital or hospice if necessary. It is best to complain as soon as possible – certainly within six months.

If you have been treated by the NHS and feel your complaint still hasn't been dealt with and you wish to make a formal complaint, there are three stages.

**Stage one: Local Resolution.** This is done through the Complaints Officer at the hospital. PALS will help you draft a letter and, if you agree, can arrange a meeting to try to resolve matters as quickly as possible. If you still aren't happy, the Complaints Manager can carry out further investigations on your behalf.

**Stage two: Independent Review.** There should be an Independent Convenor in your area who can review your complaint. The Complaints Officer or PALS can give you the address. The Convenor can ask the Complaints Manager to re-investigate, and where necessary can set up an Independent Review Panel to try to resolve your concerns. The panel will talk to all concerned and produce a short report which will be sent to you and the hospital's Chief Executive.

**Stage three: The Ombudsman.** If you still aren't happy, you can take your case to the Ombudsman (Health Service Commissioner). This is an independent person appointed by Parliament. For details, write to: The Health Service Commissioner for England, 11th Floor, Millbank Tower, London SW1P 4QP, Tel 0845 015 4033.

You can get more information about making a complaint by phoning NHS Direct on 0845 4647 or checking the website on www.nhs.direct.nhs.uk

If you have been treated privately, you should refer to your hospital's complaints procedure.

### Questions to consider
- Who are you complaining about?
- Where do they work?
- Who do they work for?
- What are you complaining about?
- When did it happen?
- What are your main concerns?
- What do you hope to achieve from making a complaint? An apology? An explanation? Action to put things right? Compensation?

### Will this affect any further treatment I might have?
Your views are important to those providing your healthcare. It is only by knowing what they are that services can be tailored to the needs of patients. It is your right to complain if you feel you have been treated poorly or unfairly, and you should never be afraid that it will affect your treatment or the services you can expect.

# Frequently heard 'facts'

**Breast cancer is the most common kind of cancer affecting women in the UK.**
*True*
Breast cancer accounts for one in four of all cancers in women.

**Antiperspirants and deodorants can cause breast cancer.**
*False*
Experts say there is no evidence for this. The reason for the increase in breast cancer seen in recent years, which is often cited as evidence, is, they say, due to the introduction of the NHS screening programme, which means more tumours are now being detected at an earlier stage in the 50–64 age group. Breast cancer is also more common as we get older, so it stands to reason that there will be more cases because of an ageing population.

**People who are left-handed are more likely to get breast cancer.**
*True*
The suggestion is that exposure of the unborn baby in the womb to steroid hormones, which influence whether you are left- or right-handed, may play a role in the development of breast cancer.

**Virgins and nuns are more likely to get breast cancer.**
*True*
The reason is that virgins and nuns don't have children, and breast cancer is closely linked to lifetime exposure to oestrogen (see p.12).

**Breast cancer is the most common reason for women to die from cancer.**
*False*
Recently lung cancer has overtaken breast cancer as the most common cancer for UK women to die from, despite the fact that breast cancer is more commonly diagnosed according to Cancer Research UK.

**More young women are dying of breast cancer.**

*False*

Death rates from breast cancer have dropped by 30 per cent in younger and middle-aged women, mainly due to the introduction of tamoxifen, which is highly effective in preventing recurrence.

**Pain is a common symptom of breast cancer.**

*False*

A painful lump is the main symptom in just 20 per cent of women with breast cancer.

**A blow on the breast or a fall can cause breast cancer.**

*False*

Trauma cannot cause breast cancer. However, a blow or a fall may accidentally draw a woman's attention to a symptom such as a lump or thickening.

**Women who are overweight are more likely to develop breast cancer.**

*Possibly true*

A growing number of studies suggest that putting on weight after the menopause may contribute to a greater risk of breast cancer – probably because fat cells are a source of oestrogen.

**Breast cancer is like blue eyes and blonde hair; you inherit it from your parents.**

*True in some cases but mostly false*

Women with a mutation in one of the breast cancer genes have an 85 per cent risk of developing breast cancer by the age of 70. However, not all will. Scientists now think that there may be a number of other common genes which many people possess that together push up the risk, but it's not as straightforward as inheriting blue eyes or blonde hair. In all cases of breast cancer, genes and environment interact.

**You're more likely to die of breast cancer in the UK than in Europe or the US.**

*Sadly this is probably true*

According to the UKBCC (United Kingdom Breast Cancer Coalition), on average 66 per cent of women in the UK are likely to be cancer free five years after diagnosis, compared with 72 per cent in Europe and 85 per cent in the US. This may be to do with longer waiting times from diagnosis to treatment and shortages of specialists and equipment in this country. In this case, figures should change with improvements in the health service.

**Survival rates vary across the country.**

*True*

If you live in Doncaster, for example, your chance of surviving five years is 69 per cent compared with 84 per cent if you live in Croydon. Generally, poorer survival rates are associated with poorer areas of the country, which may reflect later diagnosis or poorer medical services in these areas. Hopefully these inequalities should be ironed out as the National Cancer Plan is instituted in all hospitals.

**Poor women are more likely to develop breast cancer.**

*False*

In fact breast cancer tends to affect affluent women more often – possibly as a result of dietary or other factors – although poorer women are more likely to die of the disease, possibly due to lack of education and poorer access to healthcare provision.

# Breast clinics and screening units

# How to compare services

In this section of the book we list details of breast cancer services throughout the UK, organised by Cancer Network (see p.133). These are listed first for hospitals with a symptomatic breast clinic, followed by breast screening unit data.

## Mastectomy and lumpectomy volumes/waiting times

These figures are derived from Hospital Episode Statistics for the year to March 2001 and relate to NHS Trusts in England, not individual hospitals, and therefore reflect the service provided by all hospitals within that Trust. The number of procedures performed relate to patients with a primary diagnosis of breast cancer. Waiting times are median times in days from the decision to operate. Where Trust level data was not available or not applicable, '-'appears.

## % patients provided with written information

This indicates the proportion of patients who received printed or written information about their condition and/or treatment during their first appointment.

## % patients provided with support group information

This indicates the proportion of patients who were told about a support or self-help group relating to their condition before they left the hospital after their first treatment.

Both the figures above are taken from the National Survey of NHS Patients with breast cancer, one of six surveys designed to contribute to the monitoring of NHS performance from the patient's perspective. Responses relate to treatment received between July 1999 and June 2000. As above, data was collected at Trust level and applied at hospital level to indicate the information available to patients. It may be useful to consider this before your first visit to the clinic or during your first treatment, to ensure you receive the information required to help you understand your condition or treatment. Please note that where Trust level data was not available or not applicable, '-' appears.

## Additional information

A list of hospitals and other centres to which patients are referred for treatment, together with the names of reconstructive and specialist breast surgeons is provided (where this information was returned).

## Screening interval

Currently all women in the UK aged between 50 and 64 are invited for screening every 36 months. Units were asked to provide their screening interval as at 31/03/02 (if this information was not available, the number of months taken to screen 90% of the eligible screening population was provided). This data can indicate the level of available resources and the unit's efficiency, although slight differences in the reporting of this data should be considered when comparing units.

## Pre-operative diagnosis rate

This is the percentage of patients given a definite diagnosis by core biopsy or cytology before surgery. It should be borne in mind that it is not always possible to provide a pre-operative diagnosis for some breast problems, but ideally as many patients as possible should have a clear diagnosis before surgery. The National Cancer Screening programme sets a minimum standard of 70%, and a target rate of 90%.

## Small cancer detection rate

A measure of the success of the unit at detecting cancer in its early stages, this is the number of small invasive cancers (those less than 15mm in diameter) detected per 1,000 patients screened. The National Screening programme minimum standard is between 1.5 and 1.65, with the target rate between 2.0 and 2.2.

## SDR – Standardised cancer Detection Rate

The SDR is a guide to the success of a screening unit. It is the ratio of observed to expected cancers in women aged 50–64 years. The Government's minimum standard is 0.75 and the target is 1.00. An SDR of 1.00 would indicate that a unit had detected the number of cancers that it was expected to. Rates higher than one indicate that more cancers were detected than expected, and vice versa.

## Private hospital index

We tell you which private hospitals offer the core cancer services of chemotherapy, radiography and palliative care and which of these have a BUPA approved breast unit. Private hospitals usually offer surgical treatment of a wide variety of cancers, however not all of them offer radiotherapy and chemotherapy. Some patients prefer to receive the more expensive treatments under the NHS, whilst others will want to be able to receive all their treatment at one hospital, so we tell you which private hospitals can provide these treatments.

This tells you whether your hospital offers radiotherapy.

This tells you whether your hospital offers chemotherapy.

This tells you whether your hospital offers palliative care.

This tells you whether your hospital has a BUPA approved breast cancer unit.

BUPA accreditation of breast units is linked to specific specialist consultants at that hospital, and their results are regularly submitted for audit. There may be other consultants performing sugery who are not linked to the accreditation process, so it is advisable to check the list of approved consultants directly with BUPA. The unit must also be able to provide a seamless transition between all stages of treatment and if the hospital does not have all the necessary facilities it must have arrangements in place with other local hospitals that do. Listed below each hospital are the major insurers that accredit the hospital for treatment. If the insurer's name is asterisked, then they recognise that hospital as a network member and it may offer you reduced rates for treatment.

## Suvival rate table

Cancer survival is a key NHS indicator of the effectiveness of cancer treatment. Survival rates are available for England and Scotland and are calculated from the actual five year survival rate of breast cancer patients, measured against the expected survival rate if the group had the same overall mortality rate as the general population.

# Cancer Networks by region

Below is a list of UK regions, related Cancer Networks and towns within these networks.

## East
**Mid Anglia** Colchester, Ipswich **191**
**Mount Vernon** Luton, Stevenage, Watford, Welwyn Garden City **194**
**Norfolk and Waveney** Great Yarmouth, Norwich **197**
**South Essex** Basildon, Westcliff on Sea **221**
**West Anglia** Bedford, Bury St Edmunds, Cambridge, Epping, Harlow, Huntingdon, King's Lynn, Peterborough **231**

## London
**Mount Vernon** Barnet, Harrow, Uxbridge **194**
**North London 201**
**North East London 198**
**South East London 219**
**South West London 222**
**West London 235**

## North
**Humber and Yorkshire Coast** Cottingham, Scarborough **177**
**Northern** Ashington, Dryburn, Gateshead, Hexham, Newcastle upon Tyne, North Shields, South Shields, Sunderland **209**
**Teeside, South Durham and North Yorkshire** Bishop Auckland, Darlington, Hartlepool, Northallerton, Stockton on Tees **227**
**Yorkshire** Bradford, Dewsbury, Halifax, Harrogate, Huddersfield, Leeds, Steeton, Wakefield, York **238**

## North West
**Greater Manchester and Cheshire** Ashton under Lyne, Bolton, Bury, Crewe, Macclesfield, Manchester, Rochdale, Stockport, Wigan **171**
**Lancashire and South Cumbria** Barrow in Furness, Blackburn, Blackpool, Burnley, Chorley, Kendal, Lancaster, Preston **182**
**Merseyside and Cheshire** Chester, Liverpool, Ormskirk, Prescot, Runcorn, Warrington, Wirral **187**

## South East
**Central South Coast** Basingstoke, Chicester, Newport, Southampton, Winchester **158**
**Four Counties** Aylesbury, Headington, High Wycombe, Kettering,

Milton Keynes, Northampton, Oxford, Reading **166**
**Kent and Medway** Asford, Cantebury, Dartford, Gillingham, Maidstone, Margate, Tunbridge Wells **179**
**Surrey, West Sussex and Hampshire** Ashford, Guilford, Farnham **224**
**Sussex** Brighton, Worthing **226**

## South West
**Avon, Somerset and Wiltshire** Bath, Bristol, Swindon, Taunton, Yeovil **153**
**Central South Coast** Salisbury **158**
**Dorset** Bournemouth, Dorchester, Poole **164**
**Four Counties** Swindon **166**
**Peninsular** Barnstaple, Exeter, Plymouth, Torquay, Truro **217**
**Three Counties** Cheltenham, Gloucester, Stroud **229**

## Trent
**Derby and Burton** Derby **162**
**Humber and Yorkshire Coast** Boston, Lincoln **177**
**Leicestershire** Leicester **186**
**Mid Trent** Nottingham, Sutton-in-Ashfield **192**
**North Trent** Barnsley, Chesterfield, Doncaster, Rotherham, Sheffield **204**

## West Midlands
**Arden** Coventry, Nuneaton, Redditch, Warwick **151**
**Black Country** Stourbridge, Walsall, Wolverhampton **156**
**Derby and Burton** Burton upon Trent **162**
**North West Midlands** Shrewsbury, Stafford, Stoke on Trent, Telford **207**
**Pan Birmingham** Birmingham, Solihull, Sutton Coldfield, Walsall, West Bromwich, Worcester **213**
**Three Counties** Hereford, Worcester **229**

## Wales
**North and Mid Wales** Clwyd, Gwynedd, Wrexham **242**
**South East Wales** Cardiff, Ceredigion, Llantrisant, Newport **243**
**South West Wales** Bridgend, Haverfordwest, Llanelli, Swansea **244**

## Scotland
**North of Scotland** Aberdeen **245**
**South East of Scotland** Dunfermline, Edinburgh, Melrose **245**
**West of Scotland** Greenock **246**

## Northern Ireland
Currently no cancer networks exist **247**
Further information can be found at www.cancercareireland.com.

# Arden Cancer Network

### Alexandra Hospital
Woodrow Drive, Redditch, Worcestershire B98 7UB
Tel 01527 503 030

| | |
|---|---|
| Mastectomies performed | 149 |
| Mastectomy wait in days | 14 |
| Lumpectomies performed | 71 |
| Lumpectomy wait in days | 9 |

*% of patients provided with*
| | |
|---|---|
| written information | 49% |
| support group information | 75% |

### George Eliot Hospital
College Street, Nuneaton, Warwickshire CV10 7DJ
Tel 024 7635 1351

| | |
|---|---|
| Mastectomies performed | 41 |
| Mastectomy wait in days | 11 |
| Lumpectomies performed | 9 |
| Lumpectomy wait in days | 7 |

*% of patients provided with*
| | |
|---|---|
| written information | 53% |
| support group information | 69% |

**Patients referred to:**
University Hospitals Coventry and Warwickshire for complex
chemotherapy and radiotherapy

### Walsgrave Hospital
Clifford Bridge Road, Walsgrave, Coventry CV2 2DX
Tel 024 7660 2020

| | |
|---|---|
| Mastectomies performed | 129 |
| Mastectomy wait in days | 13 |
| Lumpectomies performed | 5 |
| Lumpectomy wait in days | 11 |

*% of patients provided with*
| | |
|---|---|
| written information | 58% |
| support group information | 81% |

### Warwick Hospital
Lakin Road, Warwick, Warwickshire CV34 5BW
Tel 01926 495 321

| | |
|---|---|
| Mastectomies performed | 99 |
| Mastectomy wait in days | 11 |
| Lumpectomies performed | 11 |
| Lumpectomy wait in days | 19 |

*% of patients provided with*
written information          68%
support group information    76%

**Breast surgeons:**
Mr Anthony Johnston, Mr Simon Harries

**Patients referred to:**
Coventry and Warwickshire Hospital for radiotherapy
Oncology Department at University Hospitals Coventry & Warwickshire
NHS Trust for chemotherapy
Surgery available on site

---

**Warwickshire, Solihull and Coventry BSU**
Coventry and Warwickshire Hospital
Stoney Stanton Road, Coventry CV1 4FH
Tel **024 7622 4055**

Patients are currently screened within 36 months

|                                |      |     | *98/9* | *99/0* | *00/1* |
|--------------------------------|------|-----|--------|--------|--------|
| Pre-operative diagnosis rate   | 78%  |     |        |        |        |
| Small cancer detection rate    | 2.9  | SDR | 1.01   | 1.07   | 1.21   |

---

# Avon, Somerset and Wiltshire Cancer Network

## Bristol Royal Infirmary
Marlborough Street, Bristol BS2 8HW
Tel **0117 923 0000**

| | |
|---|---|
| Mastectomies performed | 87 |
| Mastectomy wait in days | 15 |
| Lumpectomies performed | 28 |
| Lumpectomy wait in days | 12.5 |

*% of patients provided with*
| | |
|---|---|
| written information | 64% |
| support group information | 73% |

**Breast surgeons:**
Mr Z Rayter, Miss Z E Winters

**Patients referred to:**
Avon Breast Screening Centre

## Frenchay Hospital
Beckspool Road, Frenchay, Bristol BS16 1JE
Tel **0117 970 1070**

| | |
|---|---|
| Mastectomies performed | 78 |
| Mastectomy wait in days | 8 |
| Lumpectomies performed | 26 |
| Lumpectomy wait in days | 6.5 |

*% of patients provided with*
| | |
|---|---|
| written information | 76% |
| support group information | 82% |

**Breast surgeons:**
Mr S J Cawthorne, Mr A K Sahu

**Patients referred to:**
Bristol Oncology Centre for radiotherapy

## Princess Margaret Hospital
Okus Road, Swindon, Wiltshire SN1 4JU
Tel **01793 536 231**

| | |
|---|---|
| Mastectomies performed | 47 |
| Mastectomy wait in days | 20 |
| Lumpectomies performed | 28 |
| Lumpectomy wait in days | 18.5 |

*% of patients provided with*
| | |
|---|---|
| written information | 52% |
| support group information | 64% |

**Patients referred to:**
Churchill Hospital for radiotherapy, access to 'cool cap' facility
and lymphoedema clinic care
Prospect Hospice for palliative care

## Royal United Hospital
Combe Park, Bath, Somerset BA1 3NG
Tel **01225 428 331**

| | |
|---|---|
| Mastectomies performed | 112 |
| Mastectomy wait in days | 13 |
| Lumpectomies performed | 4 |
| Lumpectomy wait in days | 22.5 |

*% of patients provided with*
| | |
|---|---|
| written information | 68% |
| support group information | 81% |

**Patients referred to:**
Bristol Royal Infirmary for MRI
Frenchay Hospital for breast reconstruction

## Taunton and Somerset Hospital
Musgrove Park, Taunton, Somerset TA1 5DA
Tel **01823 333 444**

| | |
|---|---|
| Mastectomies performed | 47 |
| Mastectomy wait in days | 25 |
| Lumpectomies performed | 29 |
| Lumpectomy wait in days | 28 |

*% of patients provided with*
| | |
|---|---|
| written information | 62% |
| support group information | 74% |

## Weston General Hospital
Grange Road, Weston super Mare, Somerset BS23 4TQ
Tel **01934 636 363**

| | |
|---|---|
| Mastectomies performed | 36 |
| Mastectomy wait in days | 16 |
| Lumpectomies performed | 15 |
| Lumpectomy wait in days | 8 |

*% of patients provided with*
| | |
|---|---|
| written information | 57% |
| support group information | 83% |

**Breast surgeons:**
Mr Gallegos, Mr John

**Patients referred to:**
Bristol Royal Infirmary for breast reconstruction

## Yeovil District Hospital
Higher Kingston, Yeovil, Somerset BA21 4AT
Tel 01935 475 122

| | |
|---|---|
| Mastectomies performed | 55 |
| Mastectomy wait in days | 17 |
| Lumpectomies performed | 7 |
| Lumpectomy wait in days | 22 |

*% of patients provided with*

| | |
|---|---|
| written information | 62% |
| support group information | 75% |

**Breast surgeons:**
Mr Mohammad H Niayesh, Mr Graham Payne

**Patients referred to:**
Bristol Oncology Centre for radiotherapy
Odstock Hospital for breast reconstruction

---

## Avon BSU
Bristol Royal Infirmary
Marlborough Street, Bristol BS2 8HW
Tel 0117 923 0000

Currently, 90% of patients are screened within 38 months

| | | | 98/9 | 99/0 | 00/1 |
|---|---|---|---|---|---|
| Pre-operative diagnosis rate | 92% | | | | |
| Small cancer detection rate | 2.2 | SDR | 0.98 | 1.08 | 1.18 |

## Somerset BSU
Taunton and Somerset Hospital
Musgrove Park, Taunton, Somerset TA1 5DA
Tel 01823 333 444

Currently, 90% of patients are screened within 37 months

| | | | 98/9 | 99/0 | 00/1 |
|---|---|---|---|---|---|
| Pre-operative diagnosis rate | 95% | | | | |
| Small cancer detection rate | 3.3 | SDR | 0.95 | 1.57 | 1.31 |

## Wiltshire BSU
Princess Margaret Hospital
Okus Road, Swindon, Wiltshire SN1 4JU
Tel 01793 536 231

Currently, 90% of patients are screened within 36 months

| | | | 98/9 | 99/0 | 00/1 |
|---|---|---|---|---|---|
| Pre-operative diagnosis rate | 87% | | | | |
| Small cancer detection rate | 2.3 | SDR | 1.00 | 1.11 | 1.14 |

---

# Black Country Cancer Network

### New Cross Hospital
Wednesfield Road, Wolverhampton, West Midlands WV10 0QP
Tel **01902 307 999**

| | |
|---|---|
| Mastectomies performed | 67 |
| Mastectomy wait in days | 9 |
| Lumpectomies performed | 3 |
| Lumpectomy wait in days | 14 |

*% of patients provided with*
| | |
|---|---|
| written information | 65% |
| support group information | 85% |

**Breast surgeons:**
Mr B Isgar, Ms P Matey

### Russells Hall, Wordsley, Corbett and Guest Hospitals
Wordsley Hospital, Stream Road, Stourbridge, West Midlands DY8 5QX
Tel **01384 456 111**

| | |
|---|---|
| Mastectomies performed | 78 |
| Mastectomy wait in days | 14 |
| Lumpectomies performed | 99 |
| Lumpectomy wait in days | 14 |

*% of patients provided with*
| | |
|---|---|
| written information | 61% |
| support group information | 79% |

**Breast surgeons:**
Mr M Ali, Mr R J Blunt, Mr J T Williams

**Patients referred to:**
Cancer Support in Dudley for complementary therapy
Compton Hospital for lymphoedema
New Cross Hospital for radiotherapy

---

### Dudley and Wolverhampton BSU
Russells Hall, Wordsley, Corbett and Guest Hospitals
Wordsley Hospital, Stream Road, Wordsley, Stourbridge,
West Midlands DY8 5QX
Tel **01384 456 111**

Patients are currently screened within 36 months

| | | 98/9 | 99/0 | 00/1 |
|---|---|---|---|---|
| Pre-operative diagnosis rate 95% | | | | |
| Small cancer detection rate 1.5 | SDR | 0.86 | 1.38 | 0.84 |

**Sandwell and Walsall BSU**
Manor Hospital
Moat Road, Walsall WS2 9PS
Tel **01922 721 172**

Patients are currently screened within 38 months

| | | | 98/9 | 99/0 | 00/1 |
|---|---|---|---|---|---|
| Pre-operative diagnosis rate | 87% | | | | |
| Small cancer detection rate | 2.2 | SDR | 1.32 | 1.03 | 1.41 |

# Central South Coast Cancer Network

## North Hampshire Hospital
Aldermaston Road, Basingstoke, Hampshire RG24 9NA
Tel **01256 473 202**

| | |
|---|---|
| Mastectomies performed | 25 |
| Mastectomy wait in days | 8 |
| Lumpectomies performed | 3 |
| Lumpectomy wait in days | 3 |

*% of patients provided with*
| | |
|---|---|
| written information | 74% |
| support group information | 66% |

**Breast surgeons:**
Miss M A Stebbing, Mr I Whitworthy

**Patients referred to:**
Southampton University Hospital Trust for radiotherapy

## Queen Alexandra Hospital
Southwick Hill Road, Cosham, Portsmouth, Hampshire PO6 3LY
Tel **02392 286 000**

| | |
|---|---|
| Mastectomies performed | 105 |
| Mastectomy wait in days | 13 |
| Lumpectomies performed | 24 |
| Lumpectomy wait in days | 12 |

*% of patients provided with*
| | |
|---|---|
| written information | 63% |
| support group information | 73% |

## Royal Hampshire County Hospital
Romsey Road, Winchester, Hampshire SO22 5DG
Tel **01962 863 535**

| | |
|---|---|
| Mastectomies performed | 45 |
| Mastectomy wait in days | 7 |
| Lumpectomies performed | 9 |
| Lumpectomy wait in days | 5 |

*% of patients provided with*
| | |
|---|---|
| written information | 55% |
| support group information | 71% |

**Breast surgeons:**
Ms Siobhan Laws, Mr Dick Sainsbury

**Patients referred to:**
Royal South Hants Hospital for radiotherapy

## Salisbury District Hospital
Odstock Road, Salisbury, Wiltshire SP2 8BJ
Tel **01722 336 262**

| | |
|---|---|
| Mastectomies performed | 62 |
| Mastectomy wait in days | 7 |
| Lumpectomies performed | 13 |
| Lumpectomy wait in days | 7 |

*% of patients provided with*
written information       73%
support group information       77%

**Breast surgeons:**
A Aertssen, N J Carty

**Patients referred to:**
Poole Hospital for radiotherapy
Royal South Hants Hospital for radiotherapy
Royal United Hospital for radiotherapy

## Southampton General Hospital
Tremona Road, Southampton, Hampshire SO16 6YD
Tel **02380 777 222**

| | |
|---|---|
| Mastectomies performed | 104 |
| Mastectomy wait in days | 21 |
| Lumpectomies performed | 14 |
| Lumpectomy wait in days | 16 |

*% of patients provided with*
written information       69%
support group information       77%

**Breast surgeons:**
Mr R Allsopp, Mr E Annas, Mr J Hobby, Mr D A Rew, Mr G T Royle,
Mr I Whitworth

## St Mary's Hospital, Portsmouth
Milton Road, Portsmouth, Hampshire PO3 6AD
Tel **02392 286 000**

| | |
|---|---|
| Mastectomies performed | 105 |
| Mastectomy wait in days | 13 |
| Lumpectomies performed | 24 |
| Lumpectomy wait in days | 12 |

*% of patients provided with*
written information       63%
support group information       73%

## St Mary's Hospital, Isle of Wight
Parkhurst Road, Newport, Isle of Wight PO30 5TG
Tel **01983 524 081**

| | |
|---|---|
| Mastectomies performed | 35 |
| Mastectomy wait in days | 7 |
| Lumpectomies performed | 16 |
| Lumpectomy wait in days | 7 |

*% of patients provided with*
| | |
|---|---|
| written information | 55% |
| support group information | 72% |

**Breast surgeons:**
Mr M Shinkfield, Mr J M Symes

**Patients referred to:**
Southampton University Hospital Trust for radiotherapy
St Mary's Hospital for chemotherapy

## St Richard's Hospital
Spitalfield Lane, Chichester, West Sussex PO19 4SE
Tel **01243 788 122**

| | |
|---|---|
| Mastectomies performed | 40 |
| Mastectomy wait in days | 15 |
| Lumpectomies performed | 38 |
| Lumpectomy wait in days | 16 |

*% of patients provided with*
| | |
|---|---|
| written information | 38% |
| support group information | 67% |

**Patients referred to:**
St Mary's Hospital for oncology services

---

## Basingstoke BSU
North Hampshire Hospital
Aldermaston Road, Basingstoke, Hampshire RG24 9NA
Tel **01256 473 202**

Patients are currently screened within 34.5 months

| | | 98/9 | 99/0 | 00/1 |
|---|---|---|---|---|
| Pre-operative diagnosis rate | 71% | | | |
| Small cancer detection rate | 2.0 | SDR 1.30 | 0.72 | 1.10 |

**Winchester BSU**
Royal Hampshire County Hospital
Romsey Road, Winchester, Hampshire SO22 5DG
Tel **01962 863 535**

Patients are currently screened within 37 months

Pre-operative diagnosis rate  74%              *98/9-00/01*
Small cancer detection rate   2.0          SDR    1.12

# Derby and Burton Cancer Network

## Derby City General Hospital
Uttoxeter Road, Derby, Derbyshire DE22 3NE
Tel 01332 340 131

| | |
|---|---|
| Mastectomies performed | 164 |
| Mastectomy wait in days | 12 |
| Lumpectomies performed | 15 |
| Lumpectomy wait in days | 13 |

*% of patients provided with*
| | |
|---|---|
| written information | 77% |
| support group information | 80% |

**Breast surgeons:**
Mr H Holliday, Mr M Sibbering, Mr Y Wahedna

## Queen's Hospital
Belvedere Road, Burton upon Trent, Straffordshire DE13 0RB
Tel 01283 566 333

| | |
|---|---|
| Mastectomies performed | 15 |
| Mastectomy wait in days | 7.5 |
| Lumpectomies performed | 121 |
| Lumpectomy wait in days | 13.5 |

*% of patients provided with*
| | |
|---|---|
| written information | 77% |
| support group information | 80% |

**Breast surgeons:**
Mr T Bucknall, Mr C Rogers

**Patients referred to:**
Derby Royal Infirmary for radiotherapy
Queen Elizabeth Hospital (Birmingham) for radiotherapy

---

## South East Staffordshire BSU
Queen's Hospital
Belvedere Road, Burton upon Trent, Staffordshire DE13 0RB
Tel 01283 566 333

Patients are currently screened within 36 months

| | | | 98/9 | 99/0 | 00/1 |
|---|---|---|---|---|---|
| Pre-operative diagnosis rate | 94% | | | | |
| Small cancer detection rate | 2.2 | SDR | 0.84 | 0.56 | 0.94 |

## South Derbyshire BSU

Derby City General Hospital
Uttoxeter Road, Derby, Derbyshire DE22 3NE
Tel 01332 340 131

Patients are currently screened within 36 months

| | | 98/9 | 99/0 | 00/1 |
|---|---|---|---|---|
| Pre-operative diagnosis rate 91% | | | | |
| Small cancer detection rate 3.8 | SDR | 1.11 | 1.22 | 1.65 |

# Dorset Cancer Network

## Dorset County Hospital
Williams Avenue, Dorchester, Dorset DT1 2JY
Tel 01305 251 150

| | |
|---|---|
| Mastectomies performed | 50 |
| Mastectomy wait in days | 14 |
| Lumpectomies performed | 38 |
| Lumpectomy wait in days | 11.5 |

*% of patients provided with*
| | |
|---|---|
| written information | 62% |
| support group information | 87% |

## Poole Hospital
Longfleet Road, Poole, Dorset BH15 2JB
Tel 01202 665 511

| | |
|---|---|
| Mastectomies performed | 42 |
| Mastectomy wait in days | 16 |
| Lumpectomies performed | 46 |
| Lumpectomy wait in days | 17 |

*% of patients provided with*
| | |
|---|---|
| written information | 72% |
| support group information | 82% |

**Breast surgeons:**
Miss A A Evans, Mr J A Pain

## Royal Bournemouth Hospital
Castle Lane East, Bournemouth, Dorset BH7 7DW
Tel 01202 303 626

| | |
|---|---|
| Mastectomies performed | 59 |
| Mastectomy wait in days | 13 |
| Lumpectomies performed | 13 |
| Lumpectomy wait in days | 12 |

*% of patients provided with*
| | |
|---|---|
| written information | 66% |
| support group information | 82% |

**Breast surgeons:**
Mr A Skene, Mr S Weight

**Patients referred to:**
Lewis Manning Centre for lymphoedema
Poole General Hospital Trust for radiotherapy

**Dorset BSU**
Poole Hospital
Longfleet Road, Poole, Dorset BH15 2JB
Tel **01202 665 511**

Currently, 90% of patients are screened within 36 months

| | | | *98/9* | *99/0* | *00/1* |
|---|---|---|---|---|---|
| Pre-operative diagnosis rate | 85% | | | | |
| Small cancer detection rate | 3.0 | SDR | 1.03 | 1.15 | 1.23 |

# Four Counties Cancer Network

## Churchill Hospital
Old Road, Headington, Oxfordshire OX3 7LJ
Tel **01865 741 841**

Mastectomies performed     124
Mastectomy wait in days     4
Lumpectomies performed     40
Lumpectomy wait in days     8

*% of patients provided with*
written information     57%
support group information     75%

**Breast surgeons:**
Jane Clark, Mike Greenwall

**Patients referred to:**
John Radcliffe Hospital for outpatient services

## Horton Hospital
Oxford Road, Banbury, Oxfordshire OX16 9AL
Tel **01295 275 500**

Mastectomies performed     124
Mastectomy wait in days     4
Lumpectomies performed     40
Lumpectomy wait in days     8

*% of patients provided with*
written information     57%
support group information     75%

**Breast surgeons:**
Najam Dehalvi, Carl Griffiths

**Patients referred to:**
Churchill Hospital for radiotherapy

## John Radcliffe Hospital
Headley Way, Headington, Oxfordshire OX3 9DU
Tel **01865 741 166**

Mastectomies performed     124
Mastectomy wait in days     4
Lumpectomies performed     40
Lumpectomy wait in days     8

*% of patients provided with*
written information     57%
support group information     75%

## Kettering General Hospital

Rothwell Road, Kettering, Northamptonshire NN16 8UZ
Tel 01536 492 000

| | |
|---|---|
| Mastectomies performed | 60 |
| Mastectomy wait in days | 25 |
| Lumpectomies performed | 5 |
| Lumpectomy wait in days | 19 |

*% of patients provided with*
| | |
|---|---|
| written information | 74% |
| support group information | 58% |

**Breast surgeons:**
Mr M Rashed, Mr R D Stewart

**Patients referred to:**
Leicester Royal Infirmary for breast reconstruction
Nottingham City Hospital for breast reconstruction

## Milton Keynes General NHS Hospital

Standing Way, Milton Keynes, Buckinghamshire MK6 5LD
Tel 01908 660 033

| | |
|---|---|
| Mastectomies performed | 40 |
| Mastectomy wait in days | 9.5 |
| Lumpectomies performed | 4 |
| Lumpectomy wait in days | 19.5 |

*% of patients provided with*
| | |
|---|---|
| written information | 71% |
| support group information | 82% |

**Patients referred to:**
Northampton General Hospital for radiotherapy and chemotherapy
Oxford Radcliffe Infirmary for plastic surgery

## Northampton General Hospital

Cliftonville, Northampton, Northamptonshire NN1 5BD
Tel 01604 634 700

| | |
|---|---|
| Mastectomies performed | 73 |
| Mastectomy wait in days | 13 |
| Lumpectomies performed | 11 |
| Lumpectomy wait in days | 10 |

*% of patients provided with*
| | |
|---|---|
| written information | 59% |
| support group information | 63% |

## Princess Margaret Hospital

Okus Road, Swindon, Wiltshire SN1 4JU
Tel 01793 536 231

| | |
|---|---|
| Mastectomies performed | 47 |
| Mastectomy wait in days | 20 |
| Lumpectomies performed | 28 |
| Lumpectomy wait in days | 18.5 |

*% of patients provided with*
| | |
|---|---|
| written information | 52% |
| support group information | 64% |

**Patients referred to:**
Churchill Hospital for radiotherapy, access to 'cool cap' facility
and lymphoedema clinic care
Prospect Hospice for palliative care

## Royal Berkshire and Battle Hospital

London Road, Reading, Berkshire RG1 5AN
Tel 0118 987 5111

| | |
|---|---|
| Mastectomies performed | 53 |
| Mastectomy wait in days | 19 |
| Lumpectomies performed | 4 |
| Lumpectomy wait in days | 7 |

*% of patients provided with*
| | |
|---|---|
| written information | 54% |
| support group information | 70% |

## Stoke Mandeville Hospital

Mandeville Road, Aylesbury, Buckinghamshire HP21 8AL
Tel 01296 315 000

| | |
|---|---|
| Mastectomies performed | 44 |
| Mastectomy wait in days | 12 |
| Lumpectomies performed | 19 |
| Lumpectomy wait in days | 12 |

*% of patients provided with*
| | |
|---|---|
| written information | 64% |
| support group information | 74% |

**Breast surgeons:**
Mr Choudhray, Mr Dzumahur, Mr Taylor, Mr Tyler

**Patients referred to:**
Churchill Hospital for radiotherapy
Nightingale House Hospice for lymphoedema

## Wycombe Hospital
Queen Alexandra Road, High Wycombe, Buckinghamshire HP11 2TT
Tel 01494 526 161

| | |
|---|---|
| Mastectomies performed | 30 |
| Mastectomy wait in days | 8.5 |
| Lumpectomies performed | 92 |
| Lumpectomy wait in days | 7.5 |

*% of patients provided with*
| | |
|---|---|
| written information | 49% |
| support group information | 83% |

**Patients referred to:**
Churchill Hospital for radiotherapy
Mount Vernon Cancer Centre for radiotherapy

---

## Aylesbury BSU
Stoke Mandeville Hospital
Mandeville Road, Aylesbury, Buckinghamshire HP21 8AL
Tel 01296 315 000

Patients are currently screened within 29 months

| | | | 98/9 | 99/0 | 00/1 |
|---|---|---|---|---|---|
| Pre-operative diagnosis rate | 84% | | | | |
| Small cancer detection rate | 3.8 | SDR | 1.04 | 0.8 | 1.65 |

## East Berkshire BSU
Heatherwood Hospital
London Road, Ascot, Berkshire SL5 8AA
Tel 01753 633 000

Patients are currently screened within 34 months

| | | | 98/9 | 99/0 | 00/1 |
|---|---|---|---|---|---|
| Pre-operative diagnosis rate | 92% | | | | |
| Small cancer detection rate | 1.9 | SDR | 1.00 | 0.83 | 1.25 |

## Kettering BSU
Kettering General Hospital
Rothwell Road, Kettering, Northamptonshire NN16 8UZ
Tel 01536 492 000

Patients are currently screened within 33 months

| | | | 98/9 | 99/0 | 00/1 |
|---|---|---|---|---|---|
| Pre-operative diagnosis rate | 77% | | | | |
| Small cancer detection rate | 1.7 | SDR | 1.36 | 1.25 | 1.06 |

## Milton Keynes BSU
Milton Keynes General Hospital
Standing Way, Milton Keynes, Buckinghamshire MK6 5LD
Tel 01908 660 033

Patients are currently screened within 30 months

Pre-operative diagnosis rate 83%

| | | 98/9 | 99/0 | 00/1 |
|---|---|---|---|---|
| Small cancer detection rate | 1.8 | SDR | 0.82 | 1.25 | 1.00 |

### Northampton BSU
Northampton General Hospital
Cliftonville, Northampton, Northamptonshire NN1 5BD
Tel **01604 634 700**

Patients are currently screened within 33 months

Pre-operative diagnosis rate 96%

| | | 98/9 | 99/0 | 00/1 |
|---|---|---|---|---|
| Small cancer detection rate | 2.6 | SDR | 1.00 | 1.28 | 1.1 |

### Oxfordshire BSU
Churchill Hospital
The Old Road, Headington, Oxfordshire OX3 7LJ
Tel **01865 741 841**

Patients are currently screened within 41 months

Pre-operative diagnosis rate 93%

| | | 98/9 | 99/0 | 00/1 |
|---|---|---|---|---|
| Small cancer detection rate | 3.3 | SDR | 1.27 | 1.08 | 1.3 |

### West Berkshire BSU
Royal Berkshire and Battle Hospitals
London Road, Reading, Berkshire RG1 5AN
Tel **01189 875 111**

Due to construction problems, 74% of the patients in the last 6 months were screened within 36 months

Pre-operative diagnosis rate 88%

| | | 98/9 | 99/0 | 00/1 |
|---|---|---|---|---|
| Small cancer detection rate | 2.9 | SDR | 1.31 | 1.06 | 2.23 |

### Wiltshire BSU
Princess Margaret Hospital
Okus Road, Swindon, Wiltshire SN1 4JU
Tel **01793 536 231**

Currently, 90% of patients are screened within 36 months

Pre-operative diagnosis rate 87%

| | | 98/9 | 99/0 | 00/1 |
|---|---|---|---|---|
| Small cancer detection rate | 2.3 | SDR | 1.00 | 1.11 | 1.14 |

### Wycombe BSU
Wycombe Hospital
Queen Alexandra Road, High Wycombe, Buckinghamshire HP11 2TT
Tel **01494 526 161**

Patients are currently screened within 30 months as the unit has just moved from screening every 2 years to every 3

Pre-operative diagnosis rate 89%

| | | 98/9 | 99/0 | 00/1 |
|---|---|---|---|---|
| Small cancer detection rate | 2.3 | SDR | 1.09 | 1.38 | 1.24 |

# Greater Manchester and Cheshire Cancer Network

## Birch Hill Hospital

Union Road, Rochdale, Lancashire OL12 9QB
Tel **01706 377 777**

| | |
|---|---|
| Mastectomies performed | 27 |
| Mastectomy wait in days | 8 |
| Lumpectomies performed | 15 |
| Lumpectomy wait in days | 2 |

*% of patients provided with*
| | |
|---|---|
| written information | 68% |
| support group information | 88% |

**Breast surgeons:**
Mr I Macintosh

**Patients referred to:**
Christie Hospital for radiotherapy and chemotherapy

## Fairfield General Hospital

Rochdale Old Road, Bury, Lancashire BL9 7TD
Tel **0161 764 6081**

| | |
|---|---|
| Mastectomies performed | 32 |
| Mastectomy wait in days | 9 |
| Lumpectomies performed | 8 |
| Lumpectomy wait in days | 21 |

*% of patients provided with*
| | |
|---|---|
| written information | - |
| support group information | - |

**Breast surgeons:**
Mr M Kutiyanawala, Mr B de Sousa

**Patients referred to:**
Christie Hospital for radiotherapy

## Hope Hospital

Stott Lane, Salford, Manchester M6 8WH
Tel **0161 789 7373**

| | |
|---|---|
| Mastectomies performed | 42 |
| Mastectomy wait in days | 12 |
| Lumpectomies performed | 7 |
| Lumpectomy wait in days | 12 |

*% of patients provided with*
| | |
|---|---|
| written information | 64% |
| support group information | 76% |

## Leighton Hospital
Middlewich Road, Crewe, Lancashire CW1 4QJ
Tel **01270 255 141**

| | |
|---|---|
| Mastectomies performed | 54 |
| Mastectomy wait in days | 7 |
| Lumpectomies performed | 97 |
| Lumpectomy wait in days | 8 |

*% of patients provided with*
| | |
|---|---|
| written information | 65% |
| support group information | 85% |

**Breast surgeons:**
Mr D Cade, Mr S Selvachandran

**Patients referred to:**
Christie Hospital for radiotherapy

## Macclesfield District General Hospital
Victoria Road, Macclesfield, Cheshire SK10 3BL
Tel **01625 421 000**

| | |
|---|---|
| Mastectomies performed | 63 |
| Mastectomy wait in days | 6 |
| Lumpectomies performed | 9 |
| Lumpectomy wait in days | 6 |

*% of patients provided with*
| | |
|---|---|
| written information | 77% |
| support group information | 78% |

**Breast surgeons:**
Mr D M Matheson, Miss C Roshenlall

**Patients referred to:**
Christie Hospital for radiotherapy and some adjuvant chemotherapy

## North Manchester General Hospital
Central Drive, Crumpsall, Manchester M8 5RL
Tel **0161 795 4567**

| | |
|---|---|
| Mastectomies performed | 55 |
| Mastectomy wait in days | 6 |
| Lumpectomies performed | 12 |
| Lumpectomy wait in days | 5 |

*% of patients provided with*
| | |
|---|---|
| written information | 51% |
| support group information | 71% |

**Breast surgeons:**
Mr J M T Howat, Miss J Walls

**Patients referred to:**
Christie Hospital for radiotherapy and chemotherapy

## Royal Albert Edward Infirmary

Wigan Lane, Wigan, Lancashire WN1 2NN
Tel **01942 244 000**

| | |
|---|---|
| Mastectomies performed | 100 |
| Mastectomy wait in days | 38 |
| Lumpectomies performed | 36 |
| Lumpectomy wait in days | 28 |

*% of patients provided with*
| | |
|---|---|
| written information | 62% |
| support group information | 77% |

**Breast surgeons:**
Mr Harland

## Royal Bolton Hospital

Minerva Road, Farnworth, Bolton, Lancashire BL4 0JR
Tel **01204 390 390**

| | |
|---|---|
| Mastectomies performed | 78 |
| Mastectomy wait in days | 22 |
| Lumpectomies performed | 4 |
| Lumpectomy wait in days | 27.5 |

*% of patients provided with*
| | |
|---|---|
| written information | 51% |
| support group information | 82% |

**Breast surgeons:**
Mr Hugh M Bishop, Mr John H R Winstanley

**Patients referred to:**
Christie Hospital for radiotherapy and chemotherapy
St Mary's Hospital for genetic counselling service

## Royal Oldham Hospital

Rochdale Road, Oldham, Lancashire OL1 2JH
Tel **0161 624 0420**

| | |
|---|---|
| Mastectomies performed | 55 |
| Mastectomy wait in days | 13 |
| Lumpectomies performed | 17 |
| Lumpectomy wait in days | 11 |

*% of patients provided with*
| | |
|---|---|
| written information | 71% |
| support group information | 78% |

**Breast surgeons:**
Mr P K Luthra, Mr I H McIntosh

**Patients referred to:**
Christie Hospital for radiotherapy and some chemotherapy

## Stepping Hill Hospital

Poplar Grove, Stockport, Cheshire SK2 7JE
Tel **0161 483 1010**

| | |
|---|---|
| Mastectomies performed | 55 |
| Mastectomy wait in days | 8 |
| Lumpectomies performed | 5 |
| Lumpectomy wait in days | 6 |

*% of patients provided with*
| | |
|---|---|
| written information | 65% |
| support group information | 85% |

**Breast surgeons:**
Mr P C England

**Patients referred to:**
Central Manchester for genetic screening of high-risk patients
Christie Hospital for radiotherapy, chemotherapy and major reconstructive surgery
Wythenshawe for major reconstructive surgery
Some chemotherapy available on site

## Tameside General Hospital

Fountain Street, Ashton under Lyne, Lancashire OL6 9RW
Tel **0161 331 6000**

| | |
|---|---|
| Mastectomies performed | 39 |
| Mastectomy wait in days | 11 |
| Lumpectomies performed | 23 |
| Lumpectomy wait in days | 9 |

*% of patients provided with*
| | |
|---|---|
| written information | 72% |
| support group information | 81% |

## Trafford General Hospital

Moorside Road, Manchester M41 5SL
Tel **0161 748 4022**

| | |
|---|---|
| Mastectomies performed | 18 |
| Mastectomy wait in days | 9 |
| Lumpectomies performed | 6 |
| Lumpectomy wait in days | 5.5 |

*% of patients provided with*
| | |
|---|---|
| written information | 71% |
| support group information | 76% |

**Breast surgeons:**
Mr Al-Dabbagh

**Patients referred to:**
Christie Hospital for chemotherapy, radiotherapy, MRI or bone scan
Wythenshawe Hospital for breast reconstruction

## Wythenshawe Hospital
Southmoor Road, Wythenshawe, Manchester M23 9LT
Tel **0161 998 7070**

| | |
|---|---|
| Mastectomies performed | 102 |
| Mastectomy wait in days | 11.5 |
| Lumpectomies performed | 36 |
| Lumpectomy wait in days | 7 |

*% of patients provided with*
| | |
|---|---|
| written information | 71% |
| support group information | 80% |

---

## Bolton, Bury and Rochdale BSU
Royal Bolton Hospital
Minerva Road, Farnworth, Bolton, Lancashire BL4 0JR
Tel **01204 390 390**

Pre-operative diagnosis rate 92%
*Further information not provided*

## Crewe BSU
Leighton Hospital
Middlewich Road, Crewe, Lancashire CW1 4QJ
Tel **01270 255 141**

Patients are currently screened within 36 months

| | | 98/9 | 99/0 | 00/1 |
|---|---|---|---|---|
| Pre-operative diagnosis rate 79% | | | | |
| Small cancer detection rate 2.9 | SDR | - | - | - |

## Macclesfield BSU
Macclesfield District General Hospital
Victoria Road, Macclesfield, Cheshire SK10 3BL
Tel **01625 421 000**

Patients are currently screened within 35 months

| | | 98/9 | 99/0 | 00/1 |
|---|---|---|---|---|
| Pre-operative diagnosis rate 74% | | | | |
| Small cancer detection rate 2.5 | SDR | 1.55 | 1.00 | 0.75 |

**Wigan BSU**
Royal Albert Edward Infirmary
Wigan Lane, Wigan, Lancashire WN1 2NN
Tel **01942 244 000**

Patients are currently screened within 34 months

| | | | 98/9 | 99/0 | 00/1 |
|---|---|---|---|---|---|
| Pre-operative diagnosis rate | 80% | | | | |
| Small cancer detection rate | 2.6 | SDR | - | - | - |

# Humber and Yorkshire Coast Cancer Network

## Castle Hill Hospital
Castle Road, Cottingham, East Yorkshire HU16 5JQ
Tel **01482 875 875**

| | |
|---|---|
| Mastectomies performed | 132 |
| Mastectomy wait in days | 0 |
| Lumpectomies performed | 12 |
| Lumpectomy wait in days | 7 |

*% of patients provided with*
| | |
|---|---|
| written information | 68% |
| support group information | 71% |

## Scarborough General Hospital
Woodlands Drive, Scarborough, North Yorkshire YO12 6QL
Tel **01723 368 111**

| | |
|---|---|
| Mastectomies performed | 42 |
| Mastectomy wait in days | 6 |
| Lumpectomies performed | 7 |
| Lumpectomy wait in days | 10 |

*% of patients provided with*
| | |
|---|---|
| written information | 55% |
| support group information | 71% |

---

## Hull and East Yorkshire BSU
Castle Hill Hospital
Castle Road, Cottingham, East Yorkshire HU16 5JQ
Tel **01482 875 875**

Patients are currently screened within 36 months

| | | 98/9 | 99/0 | 00/1 |
|---|---|---|---|---|
| Pre-operative diagnosis rate | 90% | | | |
| Small cancer detection rate | 2.9 | SDR 1.55 | 1.18 | 1.51 |

## North Lincolnshire BSU
Lincoln County Hospital
Greetwell Road, Lincoln, Lincolnshire LN2 5QY
Tel **01522 512 512**

Patients are currently screened within 36 months

| | | 98/9 | 99/0 | 00/1 |
|---|---|---|---|---|
| Pre-operative diagnosis rate | 78% | | | |
| Small cancer detection rate | 1.2 | SDR 1.03 | 1.05 | 0.99 |

## South Lincolnshire BSU

Pilgrim Hospital
Sibsey Road, Boston, Lincolnshire PE21 9QS
Tel 01205 364 801

Service temporarily stopped in 2001, so patients are currently screened within 42 months

| | | | 98/9 | 99/0 | 00/1 |
|---|---|---|---|---|---|
| Pre-operative diagnosis rate | 93% | | | | |
| Small cancer detection rate | 2.4 | SDR | 1.20 | 0.93 | 1.12 |

# Kent and Medway Cancer Network

### Darent Valley Hospital
Darenth Wood Road, Dartford, Kent DA2 8DA
Tel 01322 428100

| | |
|---|---|
| Mastectomies performed | 43 |
| Mastectomy wait in days | 25 |
| Lumpectomies performed | 19 |
| Lumpectomy wait in days | 21 |

*% of patients provided with*
written information                   -
support group information        81%

### Kent and Canterbury Hospital
Ethelbert Road, Canterbury, Kent CT1 3NG
Tel 01227 766 877

| | |
|---|---|
| Mastectomies performed | 116 |
| Mastectomy wait in days | 12 |
| Lumpectomies performed | 47 |
| Lumpectomy wait in days | 13 |

*% of patients provided with*
written information                 58%
support group information        69%

### Kent and Sussex Hospital
Mount Ephraim, Tunbridge Wells, Kent TN2 4AT
Tel 01892 526 111

| | |
|---|---|
| Mastectomies performed | 76 |
| Mastectomy wait in days | 21 |
| Lumpectomies performed | 77 |
| Lumpectomy wait in days | 27 |

*% of patients provided with*
written information                 66%
support group information        72%

**Patients referred to:**
Maidstone Hospital for radiotherapy

### Maidstone Hospital
Hermitage Lane, Maidstone, Kent ME16 9QQ
Tel 01622 729 000

| | |
|---|---|
| Mastectomies performed | 76 |
| Mastectomy wait in days | 21 |
| Lumpectomies performed | 77 |
| Lumpectomy wait in days | 27 |

*% of patients provided with*
written information          66%
support group information    72%

**Patients referred to:**
East Grinstead Hospital for TRAMS reconstruction
Maidstone Hospital for radiotherapy and all other reconstructions

## Medway Maritime Hospital
Windmill Road, Gillingham, Kent ME7 5NY
Tel **01634 830 000**

Mastectomies performed       61
Mastectomy wait in days      27
Lumpectomies performed       21
Lumpectomy wait in days      23

*% of patients provided with*
written information          47%
support group information    76%

## Queen Elizabeth The Queen Mother Hospital
St Peters Road, Margate, Kent CT9 4AN
Tel **01843 225 544**

Mastectomies performed       116
Mastectomy wait in days      12
Lumpectomies performed       47
Lumpectomy wait in days      13

*% of patients provided with*
written information          58%
support group information    69%

**Patients referred to:**
Kent and Canterbury Hospital for radiotherapy and complex
chemotherapy

## William Harvey Hospital
Kennington Road, Ashford, Kent TN24 0LZ
Tel **01233 633 331**

Mastectomies performed       116
Mastectomy wait in days      12
Lumpectomies performed       47
Lumpectomy wait in days      13

*% of patients provided with*
written information          58%
support group information    69%

**Patients referred to:**
Kent and Canterbury Hospital for radiotherapy and complex
chemotherapy

**Kent BSU**
Kent and Canterbury Hospital
Ethelbert Road, Canterbury, Kent CT1 3NG
Tel 01227 766 877

Patients are currently screened within 36 months

|  |  |  | 98/9 | 99/0 | 00/1 |
|---|---|---|---|---|---|
| Pre-operative diagnosis rate | 91% |  |  |  |  |
| Small cancer detection rate | 2.8 | SDR | 1.39 | 1.22 | 1.26 |

**Kent BSU**
Medway Maritime Hospital
Windmill Road, Gillingham, Kent ME7 5NY
Tel 01634 830 000

Patients are currently screened within 36 months

|  |  |  | 98/9 | 99/0 | 00/1 |
|---|---|---|---|---|---|
| Pre-operative diagnosis rate | 90% |  |  |  |  |
| Small cancer detection rate | 2.3 | SDR | 1.11 | 1.25 | 1.21 |

**Kent BSU**
Preston Hall Hospital
London Road, Aylesford, Kent ME20 7NJ
Tel 01622 710 161

Patients are currently screened within 38 months

|  |  |  | 98/9 | 99/0 | 00/1 |
|---|---|---|---|---|---|
| Pre-operative diagnosis rate | 92% |  |  |  |  |
| Small cancer detection rate | 2.6 | SDR | 1.29 | 1.16 | 1.18 |

# Lancashire and South Cumbria Cancer Network

## Blackburn Royal Infirmary
Bolton Road, Blackburn, Lancashire BB2 3LR
Tel 01254 263 555

| | |
|---|---|
| Mastectomies performed | 60 |
| Mastectomy wait in days | 14 |
| Lumpectomies performed | 34 |
| Lumpectomy wait in days | 14 |

*% of patients provided with*
| | |
|---|---|
| written information | 71% |
| support group information | 77% |

**Breast surgeons:**
Mr J C Tresadem, Mr R J Watson

**Patients referred to:**
Blackburn, Hyndburn and Ribble Valley Healthcare NHS Trust
for breast reconstruction
Preston Cancer Centre for chemotherapy, radiotherapy and
clinical trials
Withington Hospital for breast reconstruction

## Blackpool Victoria Hospital
Whinney Heys Road, Blackpool, Lancashire FY3 8NR
Tel 01253 300 000

| | |
|---|---|
| Mastectomies performed | 65 |
| Mastectomy wait in days | 6 |
| Lumpectomies performed | 5 |
| Lumpectomy wait in days | 5.5 |

*% of patients provided with*
| | |
|---|---|
| written information | 51% |
| support group information | 74% |

## Burnley General Hospital
Casterton Avenue, Burnley, Lancashire BB10 2PQ
Tel 01282 425 071

| | |
|---|---|
| Mastectomies performed | 33 |
| Mastectomy wait in days | 12 |
| Lumpectomies performed | 18 |
| Lumpectomy wait in days | 11.5 |

*% of patients provided with*
| | |
|---|---|
| written information | 75% |
| support group information | 81% |

**Breast surgeons:**
Mr E Gross, Mr D Sandilands

**Patients referred to:**
Preston Cancer Centre for chemotherapy, radiotherapy
and clinical trials
Withington Hospital for breast reconstruction

## Chorley and South Ribble District General Hospital
Preston Road, Chorley, Lancashire PR7 1PP
Tel **01257 261 222**

| | |
|---|---|
| Mastectomies performed | 82 |
| Mastectomy wait in days | 18 |
| Lumpectomies performed | 19 |
| Lumpectomy wait in days | 21 |

*% of patients provided with*
| | |
|---|---|
| written information | 54% |
| support group information | 81% |

## Furness General Hospital
Dalton Lane, Barrow in Furness, Cumbria LA14 4LF
Tel **01229 870 870**

| | |
|---|---|
| Mastectomies performed | 108 |
| Mastectomy wait in days | 9 |
| Lumpectomies performed | 22 |
| Lumpectomy wait in days | 6 |

*% of patients provided with*
| | |
|---|---|
| written information | 65% |
| support group information | 85% |

**Breast surgeons:**
Mr J S Abraham, Mr D Allen, Mr C Ball, Miss R C Bollard,
Mr W P Morgan

**Patients referred to:**
Preston Royal Hospital for radiotherapy

## Royal Lancaster Infirmary
Ashton Road, Lancaster, Lancashire LA1 4RP
Tel **01524 659 44**

| | |
|---|---|
| Mastectomies performed | 108 |
| Mastectomy wait in days | 9 |
| Lumpectomies performed | 22 |
| Lumpectomy wait in days | 6 |

*% of patients provided with*
| | |
|---|---|
| written information | 65% |
| support group information | 85% |

**Breast surgeons:**
Mr J S Abraham, Mr D Allen, Mr C Ball, Miss R C Bollard,
Mr W P Morgan

**Patients referred to:**
Royal Preston Hospital for radiotherapy

## Royal Preston Hospital
Sharoe Green Lane North, Fulwood, Preston, Lancashire PR2 9HT
Tel **01772 716 565**

| | |
|---|---|
| Mastectomies performed | 2 |
| Mastectomy wait in days | 172 |
| Lumpectomies performed | - |
| Lumpectomy wait in days | - |

*% of patients provided with*
| | |
|---|---|
| written information | 53% |
| support group information | 67% |

## Sharoe Green Hospital
Sharoe Green Lane South, Fulwood, Preston, Lancashire PR2 8EU
Tel **01772 716 565**

| | |
|---|---|
| Mastectomies performed | 2 |
| Mastectomy wait in days | 172 |
| Lumpectomies performed | - |
| Lumpectomy wait in days | - |

*% of patients provided with*
| | |
|---|---|
| written information | 53% |
| support group information | 67% |

## Westmorland General Hospital
Burton Road, Kendal, Cumbria LA9 7RG
Tel **01539 732 288**

| | |
|---|---|
| Mastectomies performed | 108 |
| Mastectomy wait in days | 9 |
| Lumpectomies performed | 22 |
| Lumpectomy wait in days | 6 |

*% of patients provided with*
| | |
|---|---|
| written information | 65% |
| support group information | 85% |

**Breast surgeons:**
Mr J S Abraham, Mr D Allen, Mr C Ball, Miss R C Bollard,
Mr W P Morgan

**Patients referred to:**
Preston Royal Hospital for radiotherapy

## East Lancashire BSU
Accrington Victoria Hospital
Haywood Road, Accrington, Lancashire BB5 6AS
Tel **01254 263 555**

Currently, 95% of patients are screened within 36 months

| | | 98/9 | 99/0 | 00/1 |
|---|---|---|---|---|
| Pre-operative diagnosis rate 63% | | | | |
| Small cancer detection rate 3.5 | SDR | - | - | - |

## North Lancashire and South Cumbria BSU
Royal Lancaster Infirmary
Ashton Road, Lancaster, Lancashire LA1 4RP
Tel **0152 465 944**

Patients are currently screened within 37 months

| | | 98/9 | 99/0 | 00/1 |
|---|---|---|---|---|
| Pre-operative diagnosis rate 82% | | | | |
| Small cancer detection rate 2.2 | SDR | - | - | - |

# Leicestershire Cancer Network

## Glenfield Hospital
Groby Road, Leicester, Leicestershire LE3 9QP
Tel **0116 287 1471**

| | |
|---|---|
| Mastectomies performed | 161 |
| Mastectomy wait in days | 13.5 |
| Lumpectomies performed | 17 |
| Lumpectomy wait in days | 12 |

*% of patients provided with*
| | |
|---|---|
| written information | 75% |
| support group information | 82% |

## Leicester General Hospital
Gwendolen Road, Leicester, Leicestershire LE5 4PW
Tel **0116 249 0490**

| | |
|---|---|
| Mastectomies performed | 161 |
| Mastectomy wait in days | 13.5 |
| Lumpectomies performed | 17 |
| Lumpectomy wait in days | 12 |

*% of patients provided with*
| | |
|---|---|
| written information | 75% |
| support group information | 82% |

---

## Leicestershire BSU
The Breast Care Centre, Glenfield Hospital
Groby Road, Leicester, Leicestershire LE3 9QP
Tel **01162 871 471**

Patients are currently screened within 36 months

| | | | 98/9 | 99/0 | 00/1 |
|---|---|---|---|---|---|
| Pre-operative diagnosis rate 89% | | | | | |
| Small cancer detection rate 2.0 | SDR | | 1.05 | 1.08 | 1.19 |

---

# Merseyside and Cheshire Cancer Network

## Countess of Chester Hospital
Liverpool Road, Chester, Cheshire CH2 1UL
Tel 01244 365 000

| | |
|---|---|
| Mastectomies performed | 65 |
| Mastectomy wait in days | 18 |
| Lumpectomies performed | 40 |
| Lumpectomy wait in days | 14 |
| *% of patients provided with* | |
| written information | 58% |
| support group information | 66% |

**Breast surgeons:**
Mr S Dhital, Mr F Fahmy, Mrs C Harding-MacKean, Mr D McGeorge, Miss E Redmond

**Patients referred to:**
Clatterbridge Centre for Oncology for oncology services

## Halton General Hospital
Hospital Way, Runcorn, Cheshire WA7 2DA
Tel 01928 714 567

| | |
|---|---|
| Mastectomies performed | 17 |
| Mastectomy wait in days | 7 |
| Lumpectomies performed | 2 |
| Lumpectomy wait in days | 27 |
| *% of patients provided with* | |
| written information | - |
| support group information | - |

## Royal Liverpool University Hospital
Prescot Street, Liverpool L7 8XP
Tel 0151 706 2000

| | |
|---|---|
| Mastectomies performed | 204 |
| Mastectomy wait in days | 19 |
| Lumpectomies performed | 10 |
| Lumpectomy wait in days | 11.5 |
| *% of patients provided with* | |
| written information | 68% |
| support group information | 64% |

## Southport and Ormskirk Hospital NHS Trust

Ormskirk and District General Hospital
Wigan Road, Ormskirk, Lancashire L39 2AZ
Tel **01695 577 111**

Trust also delivers breast cancer services at Southport & Formby
District General Hospital

| | |
|---|---|
| Mastectomies performed | 38 |
| Mastectomy wait in days | 13 |
| Lumpectomies performed | 19 |
| Lumpectomy wait in days | 9 |

*% of patients provided with*
| | |
|---|---|
| written information | 56% |
| support group information | 87% |

**Breast surgeons:**
Mr R Alvi, Mr S Jamor, Mr S Meehan

**Patients referred to:**
Clatterbridge Centre for Oncology for radiotherapy and chemotherapy

## University Hospital Aintree

Longmoor Lane, Liverpool L9 7AL
Tel **0151 525 5980**

| | |
|---|---|
| Mastectomies performed | 45 |
| Mastectomy wait in days | 15 |
| Lumpectomies performed | 8 |
| Lumpectomy wait in days | 14.5 |

*% of patients provided with*
| | |
|---|---|
| written information | - |
| support group information | - |

**Breast surgeons:**
Mr J Dhorajiwala, Mr M Lafi, Mr L Martin

**Patients referred to:**
Clatterbridge Centre for Oncology for radiotherapy
Marie Curie Centre for lymphoedema
Woodlands Hospice Charitable Trust for complementary therapy
and lymphoedema

## Warrington Hospital

Lovely Lane, Warrington, Cheshire WA5 1QG
Tel **01925 635 911**

| | |
|---|---|
| Mastectomies performed | 44 |
| Mastectomy wait in days | 18 |
| Lumpectomies performed | 4 |
| Lumpectomy wait in days | 15 |

% of patients provided with
written information -
support group information -

## Whiston Hospital
Whiston, Prescot, Merseyside L35 5DR
Tel **0151 426 1600**

| | |
|---|---|
| Mastectomies performed | 51 |
| Mastectomy wait in days | 10 |
| Lumpectomies performed | 60 |
| Lumpectomy wait in days | 8 |

*% of patients provided with*
written information 72%
support group information 75%

**Breast surgeons:**
Mr Riccardo Audissio, Miss Leena Chagla

**Patients referred to:**
Clatterbridge Centre for Oncology for radiotherapy
Liverpool Marie Curie Centre for lymphoedema nurse specialist
Warrington General Hospital for lymphoedema nurse specialist

## Wirral Hospital (Arrowe Park and Clatterbridge)
Arrowe Park Road, Wirral, Merseyside CH49 5PE
Tel **0151 678 5111**

| | |
|---|---|
| Mastectomies performed | 52 |
| Mastectomy wait in days | 14 |
| Lumpectomies performed | 30 |
| Lumpectomy wait in days | 19 |

*% of patients provided with*
written information 74%
support group information 76%

**Breast surgeons:**
Mr D A Berstock, Mr T Y El-Sayed, Mr F M Swe

**Patients referred to:**
Clatterbridge Centre for Oncology for radiotherapy and chemotherapy

---

## Chester BSU
Countess of Chester Hospital
Liverpool Road, Chester, Cheshire CH2 1UL
Tel **01244 365 000**

Patients are currently screened within 36 months

| | | 98/9 | 99/0 | 00/1 |
|---|---|---|---|---|
| Pre-operative diagnosis rate 72% | | | | |
| Small cancer detection rate 3.2 | SDR | 1.20 | 1.70 | 1.00 |

## Liverpool BSU
Royal Liverpool University Hospital
Prescot Street, Liverpool L7 8XP
Tel **01517 062 000**

Patients are currently screened within 36 months

| | | 98/9 | 99/0 | 00/1 |
|---|---|---|---|---|
| Pre-operative diagnosis rate 82% | | | | |
| Small cancer detection rate 2.6 | SDR | - | - | - |

## Warrington, Halton, St Helens and Knowsley BSU
Warrington Hospital
Lovely Lane, Warrington, Cheshire WA5 1QG
Tel **01925 635 911**

Patients are currently screened within 34 months

| | | 98/9 | 99/0 | 00/1 |
|---|---|---|---|---|
| Pre-operative diagnosis rate 82% | | | | |
| Small cancer detection rate 2.1 | SDR | 0.70 | 0.90 | - |

## Wirral BSU
Clatterbridge Hospital
Bebington, Wirral, Merseyside L63 4JY
Tel **01513 344 000**

Patients are currently screened within 34 months

| | | 98/9 | 99/0 | 00/1 |
|---|---|---|---|---|
| Pre-operative diagnosis rate 98% | | | | |
| Small cancer detection rate 3.7 | SDR | - | - | - |

# Mid Anglia Cancer Network

**Essex County Hospital**
Lexden Road, Colchester, Essex CO3 3NB
Tel 01206 747 474

| | |
|---|---|
| Mastectomies performed | 101 |
| Mastectomy wait in days | 14 |
| Lumpectomies performed | 8 |
| Lumpectomy wait in days | 10.5 |

| *% of patients provided with* | |
|---|---|
| written information | 72% |
| support group information | 80% |

**Breast surgeons:**
Miss Fiona A MacNeill, Mr Simon K Marsh, Mr S Chandra Sekharan

---

**Chelmsford and Colchester BSU**
Essex County Hospital
Lexden Road, Colchester, Essex CO3 3NB
Tel 01206 747 474

Patients are currently screened within 39 months

| | | | *98/9* | *99/0* | *00/1* |
|---|---|---|---|---|---|
| Pre-operative diagnosis rate 87% | | | | | |
| Small cancer detection rate 2.1 | SDR | | 1.12 | 1.39 | 1.09 |

**East Suffolk BSU**
Ipswich Hospital
Heath Road, Ipswich, Suffolk IP4 5PD
Tel 01473 712 233

Patients are currently screened within 34 months

| | | | *98/9* | *99/0* | *00/1* |
|---|---|---|---|---|---|
| Pre-operative diagnosis rate 88% | | | | | |
| Small cancer detection rate 3.2 | SDR | | 0.94 | 1.36 | 1.36 |

---

# Mid Trent Cancer Network

## King's Mill Hospital
Mansfield Road, Sutton-in-Ashfield, Nottinghamshire NG17 4JL
Tel **01623 622 515**

| | |
|---|---|
| Mastectomies performed | 52 |
| Mastectomy wait in days | 9 |
| Lumpectomies performed | 60 |
| Lumpectomy wait in days | 8.5 |

*% of patients provided with*
| | |
|---|---|
| written information | 26% |
| support group information | 68% |

**Patients referred to:**
Park Hospital for private treatment

## Nottingham City Hospital
Hucknall Road, Nottingham, Nottinghamshire NG5 1PB
Tel **0115 969 1169**

| | |
|---|---|
| Mastectomies performed | 234 |
| Mastectomy wait in days | 18 |
| Lumpectomies performed | 19 |
| Lumpectomy wait in days | 15 |

*% of patients provided with*
| | |
|---|---|
| written information | 63% |
| support group information | 76% |

**Breast surgeons:**
Kwok Leung Cheung, Douglas Macmillan, John Robertson

**Patients referred to:**
Chemotherapy and radiotherapy available on site

---

## North Nottinghamshire BSU
King's Mill Hospital
Mansfield Road, Sutton-in-Ashfield, Nottinghamshire NG17 4JL
Tel **01623 622 515**

Patients are currently screened within 38 months

| | | | 98/9 | 99/0 | 00/1 |
|---|---|---|---|---|---|
| Pre-operative diagnosis rate | 97% | | | | |
| Small cancer detection rate | 3.3 | SDR | 1.00 | 0.94 | 1.04 |

## Nottingham City BSU

Nottingham City Hospital
Hucknall Road, Nottingham, Nottinghamshire NG5 1PB
Tel 01159 691 169

Patients are currently screened within 36 months

| | | | 98/9 | 99/0 | 00/1 |
|---|---|---|---|---|---|
| Pre-operative diagnosis rate | 91% | | | | |
| Small cancer detection rate | 2.5 | SDR | 1.21 | 1.20 | 1.17 |

# Mount Vernon Cancer Network

## Barnet Hospital
Wellhouse Lane, Barnet, Hertfordshire EN5 3DH
Tel **020 8216 4000**

| | |
|---|---|
| Mastectomies performed | 67 |
| Mastectomy wait in days | 19 |
| Lumpectomies performed | 24 |
| Lumpectomy wait in days | 22.5 |

*% of patients provided with*
| | |
|---|---|
| written information | 55% |
| support group information | 80% |

## Hillingdon Hospital
Pield Heath Road, Uxbridge, Middlesex UB8 3NN
Tel **01895 238 282**

| | |
|---|---|
| Mastectomies performed | 35 |
| Mastectomy wait in days | 15.5 |
| Lumpectomies performed | 15 |
| Lumpectomy wait in days | 16 |

*% of patients provided with*
| | |
|---|---|
| written information | - |
| support group information | - |

**Breast surgeons:**
Mr Addie Grobbelaar (based at Mount Vernon Hospital plastic surgery unit), Mr Vahan Kaplan, Mr Christopher Kelley, Mr Brian Shoorey

**Patients referred to:**
Mount Vernon Hospital for oncology, adjuvant treatment, plastic surgery and delayed or immediate breast reconstruction

## Lister Hospital
Coreys Mill Lane, Stevenage, Hertfordshire SG1 4AB
Tel **01226 777 835**

| | |
|---|---|
| Mastectomies performed | 111 |
| Mastectomy wait in days | 11 |
| Lumpectomies performed | 44 |
| Lumpectomy wait in days | 8.5 |

*% of patients provided with*
| | |
|---|---|
| written information | 67% |
| support group information | 82% |

**Patients referred to:**
Addenbrooke's Hospital for radiotherapy and chemotherapy
Bedford Hospital for chemotherapy
Mount Vernon Hospital for radiotherapy and chemotherapy

## Luton and Dunstable Hospital
Lewsey Road, Luton, Bedfordshire LU4 0DZ
Tel **01582 491 122**

| | |
|---|---|
| Mastectomies performed | 46 |
| Mastectomy wait in days | 10.5 |
| Lumpectomies performed | 13 |
| Lumpectomy wait in days | 13 |

*% of patients provided with*
| | |
|---|---|
| written information | 67% |
| support group information | 75% |

**Breast surgeons:**
Mr M Pittam, Mr Ravichandram

**Patients referred to:**
Mount Vernon Hospital for radiotherapy

## Northwick Park Hospital
Watford Road, Harrow, Middlesex HA1 3UJ
Tel **020 8864 3232**

| | |
|---|---|
| Mastectomies performed | 43 |
| Mastectomy wait in days | 16.5 |
| Lumpectomies performed | 7 |
| Lumpectomy wait in days | 21 |

*% of patients provided with*
| | |
|---|---|
| written information | 52% |
| support group information | 71% |

## Queen Elizabeth II Hospital
Howlands, Welvyn Garden City, Hertforshire AL7 4HQ
Tel **01707 328 111**

| | |
|---|---|
| Mastectomies performed | 111 |
| Mastectomy wait in days | 11 |
| Lumpectomies performed | 42 |
| Lumpectomy wait in days | 8.5 |

*% of patients provided with*
| | |
|---|---|
| written information | 67% |
| support group information | 82% |

**Patients referred to:**
Middlesex Hospitals for radiotherapy and some chemotherapy
Mount Vernon Hospital for radiotherapy and some chemotherapy

**Watford General Hospital**
60 Vicarage Road, Watford, Hertfordshire WD1 80HB
Tel **01923 244 366**

| | |
|---|---|
| Mastectomies performed | 61 |
| Mastectomy wait in days | 20 |
| Lumpectomies performed | 22 |
| Lumpectomy wait in days | 16.5 |

*% of patients provided with*
| | |
|---|---|
| written information | 72% |
| support group information | 75% |

**Patients referred to:**
Mount Vernon Hospital for chemotherapy and radiotherapy

---

**Bedfordshire and Hertfordshire BSU**
Luton and Dunstable Hospital
Lewsey Road, Luton, Bedfordshire LU4 0DZ
Tel **01582 491 122**

Currently, 98% of patients are screened within 38 months

| | | | *98/9* | *99/0* | *00/1* |
|---|---|---|---|---|---|
| Pre-operative diagnosis rate 89% | | | | | |
| Small cancer detection rate | 2.5 | SDR | 1.30 | 1.11 | 1.10 |

**Wycombe BSU**
Wycombe Hospital
Queen Alexandra Road, High Wycombe, Buckinghamshire HP11 2TT
Tel **01494 526 161**

Patients are currently screened within 30 months as the unit has just moved from screening every 2 years to every 3

| | | | *98/9* | *99/0* | *00/1* |
|---|---|---|---|---|---|
| Pre-operative diagnosis rate 89% | | | | | |
| Small cancer detection rate | 2.3 | SDR | 1.09 | 1.38 | 1.24 |

---

# Norfolk and Waveney Cancer Network

## James Paget Hospital
Lowestoft Road, Gorleston, Great Yarmouth, Norfolk NR31 6LA
Tel **01493 452 452**

| | |
|---|---|
| Mastectomies performed | 59 |
| Mastectomy wait in days | 7 |
| Lumpectomies performed | 12 |
| Lumpectomy wait in days | 9 |
| *% of patients provided with* | |
| written information | 77% |
| support group information | 84% |

**Breast surgeons:**
Mr J Pereira, Mr H Sturzaker

**Patients referred to:**
Norfolk and Norwich University Hospitals for radiotherapy, bone scans and some chemotherapy and plastic surgery
Some chemotherapy and plastic surgery available on site

---

## Great Yarmouth and Waveney BSU
James Paget Hospital
Lowestoft Road, Gorleston, Great Yarmouth, Norfolk NR31 6LA
Tel **01493 452 452**

Patients are currently screened within 36 months

| | | | 98/9 | 99/0 | 00/1 |
|---|---|---|---|---|---|
| Pre-operative diagnosis rate | 85% | | | | |
| Small cancer detection rate | 1.5 | SDR | 0.96 | 0.84 | 0.93 |

## Norfolk and Norwich BSU
Norfolk and Norwich Hospital
Brunswick Road, Norwich, Norfolk NR1 3SR
Tel **01603 286 286**

Current screening interval not available, but 60% of eligible women were offered an appointment within 36 months of their previous screen during the last quarter of 2000/2001

| | | | 98/9 | 99/0 | 00/1 |
|---|---|---|---|---|---|
| Pre-operative diagnosis rate | 88% | | | | |
| Small cancer detection rate | 2.9 | SDR | 1.21 | 1.60 | 1.31 |

---

# North East London Cancer Network

## Harold Wood Hospital
Gubbins Lane, Romford, Essex RM3 0BE
Tel **01708 345 533**

| | |
|---|---|
| Mastectomies performed | 62 |
| Mastectomy wait in days | 33 |
| Lumpectomies performed | 40 |
| Lumpectomy wait in days | 33.5 |

*% of patients provided with*
| | |
|---|---|
| written information | 65% |
| support group information | 71% |

## Homerton Hospital
Homerton Row, London E9 6SR
Tel **020 8510 5555**

| | |
|---|---|
| Mastectomies performed | 15 |
| Mastectomy wait in days | 3 |
| Lumpectomies performed | 1 |
| Lumpectomy wait in days | 20 |

*% of patients provided with*
| | |
|---|---|
| written information | - |
| support group information | - |

**Breast surgeons:**
Mr Mahir Mahir

**Patients referred to:**
Bart's and the London NHS Trust for radiotherapy and chemotherapy
Whipps Cross University Hospital for bone scans

## King George Hospital
Barley Lane, Ilford, Essex IG3 8YB
Tel **020 8983 8000**

| | |
|---|---|
| Mastectomies performed | 23 |
| Mastectomy wait in days | 14 |
| Lumpectomies performed | 5 |
| Lumpectomy wait in days | 4 |

*% of patients provided with*
| | |
|---|---|
| written information | 62% |
| support group information | 66% |

## Newham General Hospital
Glen Road, London E13 8SL
Tel **020 7476 4000**

| | |
|---|---|
| Mastectomies performed | 22 |
| Mastectomy wait in days | 11 |
| Lumpectomies performed | 9 |
| Lumpectomy wait in days | 6 |

*% of patients provided with*
written information        -
support group information    -

**Patients referred to:**
St Bartholomew's Hospital for reconstruction

## St Bartholomew's Hospital
West Smithfield, London EC1A 7BE
Tel **020 7377 7000**

| | |
|---|---|
| Mastectomies performed | 75 |
| Mastectomy wait in days | 30 |
| Lumpectomies performed | 21 |
| Lumpectomy wait in days | 13 |

*% of patients provided with*
written information        66%
support group information    80%

**Breast surgeons:**
Mr Ram Al-Mufti, Mr R Carpenter, Ms J M Gattuso, Mr Mahir Mahir

## Whipps Cross University Hospital
Whipps Cross Road, London E11 1NR
Tel **020 8539 5522**

| | |
|---|---|
| Mastectomies performed | 42 |
| Mastectomy wait in days | 15.5 |
| Lumpectomies performed | 26 |
| Lumpectomy wait in days | 18 |

*% of patients provided with*
written information        -
support group information    -

**Patients referred to:**
Basildon NHS Trust for breast reconstruction
St Bartholomew's Hospital for radiotherapy and chemotherapy

## Barking, Havering and Redbridge BSU
Victoria Centre
Pettits Lane, Romford, Essex RM1 4HP
Tel 01708 742 281

Patients are currently screened within 36 months

|  |  |  | 98/9 | 99/0 | 00/1 |
|---|---|---|---|---|---|
| Pre-operative diagnosis rate 80% |  |  |  |  |  |
| Small cancer detection rate 2.5 | SDR | | 1.14 | 1.15 | 1.33 |

## Central and East London BSU
St Bartholomew's Hospital
West Smithfield, London EC1A 7BE
Tel 020 7601 8888

Unit covers two health authorities, average interval across these
is 35 months

|  |  |  | 98/9 | 99/0 | 00/1 |
|---|---|---|---|---|---|
| Pre-operative diagnosis rate 92% |  |  |  |  |  |
| Small cancer detection rate 2.0 | SDR | | 1.15 | 0.97 | 0.84 |

## Waltham Forest BSU
Whipps Cross University Hospital
Leytonstone, London E11 1NR
Tel 020 8539 5522

Patients are currently screened within 32 months

|  |  |  | 98/9 | 99/0 | 00/1 |
|---|---|---|---|---|---|
| Pre-operative diagnosis rate 92% |  |  |  |  |  |
| Small cancer detection rate 0.9 | SDR | | 0.89 | 1.22 | 0.79 |

# North London Cancer Network

## Chase Farm Hospital
The Ridgeway, Enfield, Middlesex EN2 8JL
Tel 020 8366 6600

| | |
|---|---|
| Mastectomies performed | 67 |
| Mastectomy wait in days | 19 |
| Lumpectomies performed | 24 |
| Lumpectomy wait in days | 22.5 |

| *% of patients provided with* | |
|---|---|
| written information | 55% |
| support group information | 80% |

**Breast surgeons:**
Mr Victor Jaffe

**Patients referred to:**
North Middlesex Hospital for radiotherapy and chemotherapy

## Middlesex and University College Hospitals
Mortimer Street, London W1T 3AA
Tel 020 7636 8333

| | |
|---|---|
| Mastectomies performed | 39 |
| Mastectomy wait in days | 14 |
| Lumpectomies performed | 2 |
| Lumpectomy wait in days | 15.5 |

| *% of patients provided with* | |
|---|---|
| written information | 47% |
| support group information | 72% |

**Breast surgeons:**
Mr Mo Keshtgar, Mr Richard Sainsbury

## North Middlesex University Hospital
Sterling Way, Edmonton, London N18 1QX
Tel 020 8887 2000

| | |
|---|---|
| Mastectomies performed | 26 |
| Mastectomy wait in days | 10.5 |
| Lumpectomies performed | 9 |
| Lumpectomy wait in days | 12 |

| *% of patients provided with* | |
|---|---|
| written information | - |
| support group information | 60% |

**Breast surgeons:**
Mrs A Athow, Mr O Fafemi, Ms N Roche

**Patients referred to:**
Royal Free Hospital for breast reconstruction
St Bartholomew's Hospital for breast reconstruction

## Royal Free Hospital
Pond Street, Hampstead, London NW3 2QG
Tel **020 7794 0500**

| | |
|---|---|
| Mastectomies performed | 34 |
| Mastectomy wait in days | 11 |
| Lumpectomies performed | 29 |
| Lumpectomy wait in days | 13 |

| *% of patients provided with* | |
|---|---|
| written information | 55% |
| support group information | 75% |

## Whittington Hospital
Highgate Hill, Archway, London N19 5NF
Tel **020 7272 3070**

| | |
|---|---|
| Mastectomies performed | 11 |
| Mastectomy wait in days | 12 |
| Lumpectomies performed | 36 |
| Lumpectomy wait in days | 7 |

| *% of patients provided with* | |
|---|---|
| written information | - |
| support group information | - |

**Breast surgeons:**
Mr Richard Sainsbury, Mr Alan Wilson

**Patients referred to:**
Royal Free Hospital for radiotherapy

---

### North Middlesex BSU
North Middlesex University Hospital
Sterling Way, Edmonton, London N18 1QX
Tel **020 8887 2000**

Patients are currently screened within 36 months

| | | | 98/9 | 99/0 | 00/1 |
|---|---|---|---|---|---|
| Pre-operative diagnosis rate | 97% | | | | |
| Small cancer detection rate | 0.8 | SDR | 0.76 | 0.69 | 1.03 |

**North of London BSU**
Edgware Community Hospital
Burnt Oak Broadway, Edgware, Middlesex HA8 0AD
Tel **020 8952 2381**

Patients are currently screened within 36 months

| | | | 98/9 | 99/0 | 00/1 |
|---|---|---|---|---|---|
| Pre-operative diagnosis rate | 90% | | | | |
| Small cancer detection rate | 2.4 | SDR | 1.04 | 1.15 | 1.02 |

# North Trent Cancer Network

## Barnsley District General Hospital
Gawber Road, Barnsley, South Yorkshire S75 2EP
Tel **01226 730 000**

| | |
|---|---|
| Mastectomies performed | 49 |
| Mastectomy wait in days | 13 |
| Lumpectomies performed | 5 |
| Lumpectomy wait in days | 13 |

*% of patients provided with*
| | |
|---|---|
| written information | 77% |
| support group information | 92% |

**Breast surgeons:**
Mr Kenogbon

## Bassetlaw District General Hospital
Kilton Hill, Worksop, Nottinghamshire S81 0BD
Tel **01909 500 990**

| | |
|---|---|
| Mastectomies performed | 87 |
| Mastectomy wait in days | 14 |
| Lumpectomies performed | 9 |
| Lumpectomy wait in days | 19 |

*% of patients provided with*
| | |
|---|---|
| written information | 57% |
| support group information | 74% |

**Patients referred to:**
Sheffield Teaching Hospitals for breast reconstruction
Weston Park Hospital for radiotherapy

## Chesterfield and North Derbyshire Royal Hospital
Chesterfield Road, Calow, Chesterfield, Derbyshire S44 5BL
Tel **01246 277 271**

| | |
|---|---|
| Mastectomies performed | 105 |
| Mastectomy wait in days | 9 |
| Lumpectomies performed | 13 |
| Lumpectomy wait in days | 9 |

*% of patients provided with*
| | |
|---|---|
| written information | 55% |
| support group information | 77% |

**Breast surgeons:**
Mr D R Chadwick, Mr S Holt

**Patients referred to:**
Northern General Hospital for breast reconstruction

## Doncaster Royal Infirmary and Montagu Hospital

Armthrope Road, Doncaster, South Yorkshire DN2 5LT
Tel 01302 366 666

| | |
|---|---|
| Mastectomies performed | 87 |
| Mastectomy wait in days | 14 |
| Lumpectomies performed | 9 |
| Lumpectomy wait in days | 19 |

*% of patients provided with*
written information 57%
support group information 74%

## Northern General Hospital

Herries Road, Sheffield, Yorkshire S5 7AU
Tel 0114 243 4343

| | |
|---|---|
| Mastectomies performed | 51 |
| Mastectomy wait in days | 16 |
| Lumpectomies performed | 8 |
| Lumpectomy wait in days | 7 |

*% of patients provided with*
written information 46%
support group information 65%

## Rotherham District General Hospital

Moorgate Road, Rotherham, South Yorkshire S60 2UD
Tel 01709 820 000

| | |
|---|---|
| Mastectomies performed | 74 |
| Mastectomy wait in days | 15 |
| Lumpectomies performed | 1 |
| Lumpectomy wait in days | 20 |

*% of patients provided with*
written information 70%
support group information 86%

---

## Barnsley BSU

Barnsley District General Hospital
Gawber Road, Barnsley, South Yorkshire S75 2EP
Tel 01226 730 000

Currently, 96% of patients are screened within 36 months

| | | 98/9 | 99/0 | 00/1 |
|---|---|---|---|---|
| Pre-operative diagnosis rate 98% | | | | |
| Small cancer detection rate 2.7 | SDR | 1.11 | 0.90 | 1.50 |

**Doncaster BSU**
Doncaster Royal Infirmary/Bassetlaw District General Hospital
Armthrope Road, Doncaster, South Yorkshire DN2 5LT
Tel 01302 366 666

Patients are currently screened within 36 months

| | | | 98/9 | 99/0 | 00/1 |
|---|---|---|---|---|---|
| Pre-operative diagnosis rate 98% | | | | | |
| Small cancer detection rate 1.6 | SDR | | 1.18 | 1.22 | 0.96 |

**North Derbyshire BSU**
Chesterfield and North Derbyshire Royal Hospital
Chesterfield Road, Calow, Chesterfield, Derbyshire S44 5BL
Tel 01246 277 271

Patients are currently screened within 36 months

| | | | 98/9 | 99/0 | 00/1 |
|---|---|---|---|---|---|
| Pre-operative diagnosis rate 94% | | | | | |
| Small cancer detection rate 2.5 | SDR | | 1.29 | 0.79 | 1.34 |

**Rotherham BSU**
Rotherham District General Hospital
Moorgate Road, Rotherham, South Yorkshire S60 2UD
Tel 01709 820 000

Patients are currently screened within 36 months

| | | | 98/9 | 99/0 | 00/1 |
|---|---|---|---|---|---|
| Pre-operative diagnosis rate 83% | | | | | |
| Small cancer detection rate 2.8 | SDR | | 1.01 | 1.07 | 1.13 |

**Sheffield BSU**
Royal Hallamshire Hospital
Glossop Road, Sheffield, Yorkshire S10 2JF
Tel 0114 271 1900

Patients are currently screened within 36 months

| | | | 98/9 | 99/0 | 00/1 |
|---|---|---|---|---|---|
| Pre-operative diagnosis rate 88% | | | | | |
| Small cancer detection rate 2.1 | SDR | | 1.04 | 1.00 | 0.99 |

# North West Midlands Cancer Network

## North Staffordshire Hospital
Royal Infirmary, Princes Road, Stoke on Trent ST4 7LN
Tel **01782 715 444**

| | |
|---|---|
| Mastectomies performed | 123 |
| Mastectomy wait in days | 12 |
| Lumpectomies performed | 27 |
| Lumpectomy wait in days | 17 |

*% of patients provided with*
| | |
|---|---|
| written information | 74% |
| support group information | 87% |

## Princess Royal Hospital
Apley Castle, Telford, Shropshire TF1 6TF
Tel **01952 641 222**

| | |
|---|---|
| Mastectomies performed | 52 |
| Mastectomy wait in days | 13 |
| Lumpectomies performed | 12 |
| Lumpectomy wait in days | 10 |

*% of patients provided with*
| | |
|---|---|
| written information | 65% |
| support group information | 70% |

**Breast surgeons:**
Mr Hinton, Mr Usman

**Patients referred to:**
Royal Shrewsbury Hospital for radiotherapy and oncology
The Hamar Centre in Shrewsbury for complementary therapy

## Royal Shrewsbury Hospital
Mytton Oak Road, Shrewsbury, Shropshire SY3 8XQ
Tel **01743 261 000**

| | |
|---|---|
| Mastectomies performed | 35 |
| Mastectomy wait in days | 12.5 |
| Lumpectomies performed | 34 |
| Lumpectomy wait in days | 16 |

*% of patients provided with*
| | |
|---|---|
| written information | 61% |
| support group information | 75% |

**Patients referred to:**
Christie Hospital for plastic surgery
North Staffordshire Hospital for plastic surgery

## Staffordshire General Hospital

Weston Road, Stafford, Staffordshire ST16 3SA
Tel 01785 257 731

| | |
|---|---|
| Mastectomies performed | 20 |
| Mastectomy wait in days | 18 |
| Lumpectomies performed | 2 |
| Lumpectomy wait in days | 26.5 |

*% of patients provided with*
| | |
|---|---|
| written information | 67% |
| support group information | 67% |

**Breast surgeons:**
Mr R Gendy, Mr B R Gwynn

**Patients referred to:**
North Staffordshire Hospital NHS Trust for radiotherapy
Royal Wolverhampton Hospitals NHS Trust for radiotherapy

---

### Mid Staffordshire BSU

Staffordshire General Hospital
Weston Road, Stafford ST16 3SA
Tel 01785 257 731

Patients are currently screened within 36 months

| | | 98/9 | 99/0 | 00/1 |
|---|---|---|---|---|
| Pre-operative diagnosis rate 88% | | | | |
| Small cancer detection rate 3.2 | SDR | 1.00 | 1.04 | 1.48 |

### North Staffordshire BSU

North Staffordshire Hospital
Royal Infirmary, Princes Road, Hartshill, Stoke on Trent ST4 7LN
Tel 01782 715 444

Patients are currently screened within 38 months

| | | 98/9 | 99/0 | 00/1 |
|---|---|---|---|---|
| Pre-operative diagnosis rate 85% | | | | |
| Small cancer detection rate 2.2 | SDR | 1.03 | 1.04 | 0.88 |

### Shropshire BSU

Royal Shrewsbury Hospital
Mytton Oak Road, Shrewsbury, Shropshire SY3 8XQ
Tel 01743 261 000

Patients are currently screened within 38 months

| | | 98/9 | 99/0 | 00/1 |
|---|---|---|---|---|
| Pre-operative diagnosis rate 94% | | | | |
| Small cancer detection rate 2.3 | SDR | 1.18 | 1.07 | 1.31 |

# Northern Cancer Network

**Freeman Hospital, Newcastle General Hospital, Royal Victoria Infirmary**
Freeman Road, High Heaton, Newcastle upon Tyne NE7 7DN
Tel **0191 284 3111**

| | |
|---|---|
| Mastectomies performed | 141 |
| Mastectomy wait in days | 0 |
| Lumpectomies performed | 105 |
| Lumpectomy wait in days | 0 |

*% of patients provided with*
| | |
|---|---|
| written information | 76% |
| support group information | 68% |

**Breast surgeons:**
Mr R Bliss, Mr A B Griffiths, Professor T W J Lennard

**Hexham General Hospital**
Corbridge Road, Hexham, Northumberland NE46 1QJ
Tel **01434 655 655**

| | |
|---|---|
| Mastectomies performed | 94 |
| Mastectomy wait in days | 9 |
| Lumpectomies performed | 18 |
| Lumpectomy wait in days | 6 |

*% of patients provided with*
| | |
|---|---|
| written information | 71% |
| support group information | 74% |

**Patients referred to:**
Newcastle Centre for Cancer Treatment (NCCT) for radiotherapy
and chemotherapy
Newcastle upon Tyne Hospitals for surgery

**North Tyneside General Hospital**
Rake Lane, North Shields, Tyne & Wear NE29 8NH
Tel **0191 259 6660**

| | |
|---|---|
| Mastectomies performed | 94 |
| Mastectomy wait in days | 9 |
| Lumpectomies performed | 18 |
| Lumpectomy wait in days | 6 |

*% of patients provided with*
| | |
|---|---|
| written information | 71% |
| support group information | 74% |

**Patients referred to:**
Newcastle Centre for Cancer Treatment (NCCT) for radiotherapy
and chemotherapy (clinical trial patients)

## Queen Elizabeth Hospital
Queen Elizabeth Avenue, Gateshead, Tyne & Wear NE9 6SX
Tel **0191 482 0000**

| | |
|---|---|
| Mastectomies performed | 124 |
| Mastectomy wait in days | 18 |
| Lumpectomies performed | 7 |
| Lumpectomy wait in days | 23 |

*% of patients provided with*
| | |
|---|---|
| written information | 70% |
| support group information | 75% |

**Breast surgeons:**
Mr Browell, Mr Cunlisse, Mr Gatehouse

**Patients referred to:**
Newcastle upon Tyne Hospitals for radiotherapy and breast reconstruction

## South Tyneside District Hospital
Harton Lane, South Shields, Tyne & Wear NE34 0PL
Tel **0191 454 8888**

| | |
|---|---|
| Mastectomies performed | 25 |
| Mastectomy wait in days | 7 |
| Lumpectomies performed | 8 |
| Lumpectomy wait in days | 7 |

*% of patients provided with*
| | |
|---|---|
| written information | - |
| support group information | - |

**Breast surgeons:**
Mr C J Pritchett (at NCCT Newcastle General)

**Patients referred to:**
Newcastle Centre for Cancer Treatment ( NCCT) for radiotherapy
University Hospital of North Durham for breast reconstruction

## Sunderland Royal Hospital
Kayll Road, Sunderland, Tyne & Wear SR4 7TP
Tel **0191 565 6256**

| | |
|---|---|
| Mastectomies performed | 67 |
| Mastectomy wait in days | 9 |
| Lumpectomies performed | 46 |
| Lumpectomy wait in days | 8 |

*% of patients provided with*
| | |
|---|---|
| written information | 75% |
| support group information | 79% |

## University Hospital of North Durham
(combined service with Shotley Bridge Hospital)
North Road, Dryburn, County Durham DH1 5TW
Tel **0191 333 2333**

| | |
|---|---|
| Mastectomies performed | 54 |
| Mastectomy wait in days | 10 |
| Lumpectomies performed | 3 |
| Lumpectomy wait in days | 13 |

*% of patients provided with*
| | |
|---|---|
| written information | 39% |
| support group information | 48% |

**Breast surgeons:**
Mr R B Berry, Mr Kevin Clark, Mr A I M Cook, Mr M W H Erdmann,
Mr G S Rao

**Patients referred to:**
Newcastle upon Tyne Hospitals for radiotherapy

## Wansbeck General Hospital
Woodhorn Lane, Ashington, Northumberland NE63 9JJ
Tel **01670 521 212**

| | |
|---|---|
| Mastectomies performed | 94 |
| Mastectomy wait in days | 9 |
| Lumpectomies performed | 18 |
| Lumpectomy wait in days | 6 |

*% of patients provided with*
| | |
|---|---|
| written information | 71% |
| support group information | 74% |

**Patients referred to:**
Newcastle Centre for Cancer Treatment ( NCCT) for radiotherapy
and chemotherapy (including clinical trial patients)
St Oswald's Hospice for lymphoedema

---

## Gateshead BSU
Queen Elizabeth Hospital
Sheriff Hill, Gateshead, Tyne & Wear NE9 6SX
Tel **01914 820 000**

Patients are currently screened within 36 months

| | | | 98/9 | 99/0 | 00/1 |
|---|---|---|---|---|---|
| Pre-operative diagnosis rate | 82% | | | | |
| Small cancer detection rate | 2.3 | SDR | 1.10 | 1.25 | 1.32 |

## Newcastle BSU

Royal Victoria Infirmary
Queen Victoria Road, Newcastle upon Tyne NE1 4LP
Tel **01912 325 131**

Patients are currently screened within 36 months

| | | | 98/9 | 99/0 | 00/1 |
|---|---|---|---|---|---|
| Pre-operative diagnosis rate | 81% | | | | |
| Small cancer detection rate | 2.1 | SDR | 1.32 | 1.14 | 1.27 |

## North Cumbria BSU

Cumberland Infirmary
Newtown Road, Carlisle, Cumbria CA2 7HY
Tel **01228 523 444**

Patients are currently screened within 36 months

| | | | 98/9 | 99/0 | 00/1 |
|---|---|---|---|---|---|
| Pre-operative diagnosis rate | 91% | | | | |
| Small cancer detection rate | 3.7 | SDR | - | - | - |

# Pan Birmingham Cancer Network

## Birmingham Heartlands Hospital
Bordesley Green East, Bordesley Green, Birmingham B9 5SS
Tel 0121 424 2000

| | |
|---|---|
| Mastectomies performed | 96 |
| Mastectomy wait in days | 13 |
| Lumpectomies performed | 14 |
| Lumpectomy wait in days | 13 |

*% of patients provided with*
| | |
|---|---|
| written information | 59% |
| support group information | 72% |

## City Hospital
Dudley Road, Winton Green, Birmingham B18 7QH
Tel 0121 554 3801

| | |
|---|---|
| Mastectomies performed | 73 |
| Mastectomy wait in days | 21 |
| Lumpectomies performed | 19 |
| Lumpectomy wait in days | 14 |

*% of patients provided with*
| | |
|---|---|
| written information | 73% |
| support group information | 87% |

## Good Hope District General Hospital
Rectory Road, Sutton Coldfield, West Midlands B75 7RR
Tel 0121 378 2211

| | |
|---|---|
| Mastectomies performed | 128 |
| Mastectomy wait in days | 11 |
| Lumpectomies performed | 12 |
| Lumpectomy wait in days | 13 |

*% of patients provided with*
| | |
|---|---|
| written information | 67% |
| support group information | 87% |

**Patients referred to:**
City Hospital for breast reconstruction
Queen Elizabeth Hospital for radiotherapy and some chemotherapy
Selly Oak Hospital for breast reconstruction

## Manor Hospital

Moat Road, Walsall WS2 9PS
Tel **01922 721 172**

| | |
|---|---|
| Mastectomies performed | 121 |
| Mastectomy wait in days | 10 |
| Lumpectomies performed | 24 |
| Lumpectomy wait in days | 11 |

*% of patients provided with*
| | |
|---|---|
| written information | 72% |
| support group information | 90% |

## Sandwell General Hospital

Lyndon, West Bromwich, West Midlands B71 4HU
Tel **0121 553 1831**

| | |
|---|---|
| Mastectomies performed | 48 |
| Mastectomy wait in days | 12 |
| Lumpectomies performed | 71 |
| Lumpectomy wait in days | 10 |

*% of patients provided with*
| | |
|---|---|
| written information | 70% |
| support group information | 81% |

**Breast surgeons:**
Mr A Aukland, Mr D Ellis

## Selly Oak Hospital

Raddlebarn Road, Birmingham B29 6JD
Tel **0121 627 1627**

| | |
|---|---|
| Mastectomies performed | 115 |
| Mastectomy wait in days | 10 |
| Lumpectomies performed | 49 |
| Lumpectomy wait in days | 7 |

*% of patients provided with*
| | |
|---|---|
| written information | 70% |
| support group information | 81% |

**Breast surgeons:**
Mr David England, Mr John Fielding, Ms Adele Francis, Mr Mike Hallissey, Ms C C Katt

## Solihull Hospital

Lode Lane, Solihull, West Midlands B91 2JL
Tel **0121 424 2000**

| | |
|---|---|
| Mastectomies performed | 96 |
| Mastectomy wait in days | 13 |
| Lumpectomies performed | 14 |
| Lumpectomy wait in days | 13 |

% of patients provided with
written information              59%
support group information       72%

## Worcester Royal Hospital
Ronkswood Branch, Newtown Road, Worcester WR5 1HN
Tel **01905 763 333**

| | |
|---|---|
| Mastectomies performed | 149 |
| Mastectomy wait in days | 14 |
| Lumpectomies performed | 71 |
| Lumpectomy wait in days | 9 |

% of patients provided with
written information              49%
support group information       75%

---

## Hereford and Worcester BSU
Princess of Wales Community Hospital
Stourbridge Road, Bromsgrove, Worcestershire B61 0BB
Tel **01527 488 000**

Patients are currently screened within 38 months

| | | | 98/9 | 99/0 | 00/1 |
|---|---|---|---|---|---|
| Pre-operative diagnosis rate | 85% | | | | |
| Small cancer detection rate | 2.1 | SDR | 1.16 | 1.14 | 0.96 |

## North Birmingham BSU
City Hospital
Dudley Road, Winton Green, Birmingham B18 7QH
Tel **01215 543 801**

Patients are currently screened within 38 months

| | | | 98/9 | 99/0 | 00/1 |
|---|---|---|---|---|---|
| Pre-operative diagnosis rate | 88% | | | | |
| Small cancer detection rate | 2.1 | SDR | 1.04 | 0.96 | 1.21 |

## Sandwell and Walsall BSU
Manor Hospital
Moat Road, Walsall WS2 9PS
Tel **01922 721 172**

Patients are currently screened within 38 months

| | | | 98/9 | 99/0 | 00/1 |
|---|---|---|---|---|---|
| Pre-operative diagnosis rate | 87% | | | | |
| Small cancer detection rate | 2.2 | SDR | 1.32 | 1.03 | 1.41 |

## South Birmingham BSU

Selly Oak Hospital
Raddlebarn Road, Birmingham B29 6JD
Tel **01216 271 627**

Patients are currently screened within 38 months

| | | 98/9 | 99/0 | 00/1 |
|---|---|---|---|---|
| Pre-operative diagnosis rate 92% | | | | |
| Small cancer detection rate 1.9 | SDR | 0.73 | 1.20 | 1.28 |

# Peninsular Cancer Network

### North Devon District Hospital
Raleigh Park, Barnstaple, Devon EX31 4JB
Tel **01271 322 577**

| | |
|---|---|
| Mastectomies performed | 48 |
| Mastectomy wait in days | 13 |
| Lumpectomies performed | 22 |
| Lumpectomy wait in days | 15 |

*% of patients provided with*
| | |
|---|---|
| written information | 54% |
| support group information | 73% |

### Royal Cornwall Hospital
Treliske, Truro, Cornwall TR1 3LJ
Tel **01872 250 000**

| | |
|---|---|
| Mastectomies performed | 112 |
| Mastectomy wait in days | 16.5 |
| Lumpectomies performed | 92 |
| Lumpectomy wait in days | 6 |

*% of patients provided with*
| | |
|---|---|
| written information | 43% |
| support group information | 55% |

**Patients referred to:**
Mount Edgecumbe Hospice for lymphoedema
Derriford Hospital for radiotherapy and breast reconstruction

### Royal Devon and Exeter Hospital
Barrack Road, Exeter, Devon EX2 5DW
Tel **01392 411 611**

| | |
|---|---|
| Mastectomies performed | 119 |
| Mastectomy wait in days | 18 |
| Lumpectomies performed | 39 |
| Lumpectomy wait in days | 23 |

*% of patients provided with*
| | |
|---|---|
| written information | 63% |
| support group information | 69% |

### Torbay District General Hospital
Lawes Bridge, Torquay, Devon TQ2 7AA
Tel **01803 614 567**

| | |
|---|---|
| Mastectomies performed | 29 |
| Mastectomy wait in days | 14 |
| Lumpectomies performed | 127 |
| Lumpectomy wait in days | 11 |

*% of patients provided with*
written information      71%
support group information      83%

**Breast surgeons:**
Mr Peter Donnelly, Mr Robin Hughes

**Patients referred to:**
Royal Devon and Exeter Hospital for breast reconstuction and
radiotherapy treatment boost with electrons

---

### Cornwall BSU

The Mermaid Centre, Royal Cornwall Hospital
Treliske, Truro, Cornwall TR1 3LJ
Tel **01872 250 000**

Patients are currently screened within 35 months

| | | | 98/9 | 99/0 | 00/1 |
|---|---|---|---|---|---|
| Pre-operative diagnosis rate 80% | | | | | |
| Small cancer detection rate   1.7 | | SDR | 1.12 | 0.99 | 0.85 |

### East Devon BSU

Royal Devon and Exeter Hospital
Barrack Road, Wonford, Exeter, Devon EX2 5DW
Tel **01392 411 611**

Patients are currently screened within 43 months

| | | | 98/9 | 99/0 | 00/1 |
|---|---|---|---|---|---|
| Pre-operative diagnosis rate 88% | | | | | |
| Small cancer detection rate   2.0 | | SDR | 1.19 | 1.40 | 1.10 |

### West Devon BSU

Derriford Hospital
Derriford Road, Plymouth, Devon PL6 8DH
Tel **01752 777 111**

Currently, 90% of patients are screened within 34 months

| | | | 98/9 | 99/0 | 00/1 |
|---|---|---|---|---|---|
| Pre-operative diagnosis rate 90% | | | | | |
| Small cancer detection rate   2.0 | | SDR | 1.43 | 1.07 | 0.84 |

---

# South East London Cancer Network

## Bromley Hospital
Cromwell Avenue, Bromley, Kent BR2 9AJ
Tel **020 8289 7000**

| | |
|---|---|
| Mastectomies performed | 36 |
| Mastectomy wait in days | 17.5 |
| Lumpectomies performed | 13 |
| Lumpectomy wait in days | 14 |

*% of patients provided with*
| | |
|---|---|
| written information | 64% |
| support group information | 72% |

**Breast surgeons:**
Mr Aluwihare, Mr Desai

**Patients referred to:**
Guy's and St Thomas' NHS Trust for radiotherapy

## Farnborough Hospital
Farnborough Common, Orpington, Kent BR6 8ND
Tel **01689 814 000**

| | |
|---|---|
| Mastectomies performed | 36 |
| Mastectomy wait in days | 17.5 |
| Lumpectomies performed | 13 |
| Lumpectomy wait in days | 14 |

*% of patients provided with*
| | |
|---|---|
| written information | 64% |
| support group information | 72% |

## King's College Hospital
Denmark Hill, London SE5 9RS
Tel **020 7737 4000**

| | |
|---|---|
| Mastectomies performed | 27 |
| Mastectomy wait in days | 19.5 |
| Lumpectomies performed | 25 |
| Lumpectomy wait in days | 19 |

*% of patients provided with*
| | |
|---|---|
| written information | 65% |
| support group information | 68% |

**Breast surgeons:**
Mr Jonathan V Roberts

## Queen Elizabeth Hospital

Stadium Road, London SE18 4QH
Tel 020 8858 8141

| | |
|---|---|
| Mastectomies performed | 37 |
| Mastectomy wait in days | 10 |
| Lumpectomies performed | 4 |
| Lumpectomy wait in days | 8.5 |

*% of patients provided with*
| | |
|---|---|
| written information | 67% |
| support group information | 73% |

**Breast surgeons:**
Mr Al-Hilaly, Mr Rather, Mr A Stoker

**Patients referred to:**
Bexley and Greenwich Hospice for lymphoedema
Genetics clinic at Guy's Hospital for genetic testing
St Thomas' Hospital for radiotherapy

## Queen Mary's Hospital

Frognal Avenue, Sidcup, Kent DA14 6LT
Tel 020 8302 2678

| | |
|---|---|
| Mastectomies performed | 23 |
| Mastectomy wait in days | 13 |
| Lumpectomies performed | 13 |
| Lumpectomy wait in days | 11 |

*% of patients provided with*
| | |
|---|---|
| written information | 63% |
| support group information | 82% |

---

## South East London BSU

King's College Hospital
Denmark Hill, London SE5 9RS
Tel 020 7737 4000

Patients are currently screened within 36 months

| | | | | 98/9 | 99/0 | 00/1 |
|---|---|---|---|---|---|---|
| Pre-operative diagnosis rate | 91% | | | | | |
| Small cancer detection rate | 2.5 | | SDR | 1.00 | 0.89 | 1.09 |

---

# South Essex Cancer Network

## Basildon Hospital
Nethermayne, Basildon, Essex SS16 5NL
Tel 01268 533 911

| | |
|---|---|
| Mastectomies performed | 17 |
| Mastectomy wait in days | 18 |
| Lumpectomies performed | 23 |
| Lumpectomy wait in days | 17 |

*% of patients provided with*
| | |
|---|---|
| written information | 61% |
| support group information | 78% |

## Southend Hospital
Prittlewell Chase, Westcliff on Sea, Essex SS0 0RT
Tel 01702 435 555

| | |
|---|---|
| Mastectomies performed | 76 |
| Mastectomy wait in days | 10 |
| Lumpectomies performed | 144 |
| Lumpectomy wait in days | 8.5 |

*% of patients provided with*
| | |
|---|---|
| written information | 60% |
| support group information | 77% |

---

## South Essex BSU
Southend Hospital
Prittlewell Chase, Westcliff on Sea, Essex SS0 0RT
Tel 01702 435 555

Patients are currently screened within 34-36 months

| | | 98/9 | 99/0 | 00/1 |
|---|---|---|---|---|
| Pre-operative diagnosis rate 88% | | | | |
| Small cancer detection rate 2.7 | SDR | 1.39 | 1.23 | 1.22 |

# South West London Cancer Network

### Kingston Hospital
Galsworthy Road, Kingston upon Thames, Surrey KT2 7QB
Tel **020 8546 7711**

| | |
|---|---|
| Mastectomies performed | 23 |
| Mastectomy wait in days | 11 |
| Lumpectomies performed | 68 |
| Lumpectomy wait in days | 12 |

*% of patients provided with*
| | |
|---|---|
| written information | - |
| support group information | 79% |

**Patients referred to:**
Charing Cross Hospital for radiotherapy, chemotherapy and breast reconstruction

### Mayday Hospital
530 London Road, Thornton Heath CR7 7YE
Tel **0208 401 3000**

| | |
|---|---|
| Mastectomies performed | 57 |
| Mastectomy wait in days | 12 |
| Lumpectomies performed | 13 |
| Lumpectomy wait in days | 18 |

*% of patients provided with*
| | |
|---|---|
| written information | 70% |
| support group information | 75% |

**Breast surgeons:**
Miss A Advani, Mr S Ebbs, Mr P Meagher, Mr J Wickers

**Patients referred to:**
Royal Marsden Hospital for radiotherapy and chemotherapy

### St George's Hospital
Blackshaw Road, London SW17 0QT
Tel **020 8672 1255**

| | |
|---|---|
| Mastectomies performed | 56 |
| Mastectomy wait in days | 20.5 |
| Lumpectomies performed | 21 |
| Lumpectomy wait in days | 15 |

*% of patients provided with*
| | |
|---|---|
| written information | 54% |
| support group information | 78% |

## South West London BSU

St George's Hospital
Blackshaw Road, London SW17 0QT
Tel **020 8672 1255**

Patients are currently screened within 42 months

| | | | 98/9 | 99/0 | 00/1 |
|---|---|---|---|---|---|
| Pre-operative diagnosis rate | 91% | | | | |
| Small cancer detection rate | 3.0 | SDR | 1.30 | 1.39 | 1.50 |

# Surrey, West Sussex and Hampshire Cancer Network

## Ashford Hospital
London Road, Ashford, Middlesex TW15 3AA
Tel **01784 884 488**

| | |
|---|---|
| Mastectomies performed | 23 |
| Mastectomy wait in days | 20 |
| Lumpectomies performed | 21 |
| Lumpectomy wait in days | 22 |

*% of patients provided with*
| | |
|---|---|
| written information | 72% |
| support group information | 76% |

## Crawley Hospital
West Green Drive, Crawley, West Sussex RH11 7DH
Tel **01293 600 300**

| | |
|---|---|
| Mastectomies performed | 44 |
| Mastectomy wait in days | 17 |
| Lumpectomies performed | 18 |
| Lumpectomy wait in days | 20 |

*% of patients provided with*
| | |
|---|---|
| written information | 59% |
| support group information | 67% |

**Breast surgeons:**
Mr A Ball, Mr A Stacey-Clear

**Patients referred to:**
Royal Surrey County Hospital for chemotherapy and radiotherapy

## Frimley Park Hospital
Portsmouth Road, Frimley, Surrey GU16 7UJ
Tel **01276 604 604**

| | |
|---|---|
| Mastectomies performed | 50 |
| Mastectomy wait in days | 13 |
| Lumpectomies performed | 4 |
| Lumpectomy wait in days | 22.5 |

*% of patients provided with*
| | |
|---|---|
| written information | 58% |
| support group information | 62% |

**Breast surgeons:**
Mr R Daoud, Mr Ian Laidlaw

**Patients referred to:**
St Luke's Cancer Centre for radiotherapy and chemotherapy

## Royal Surrey County Hospital
Egerton Road, Guildford, Surrey GU2 7XX
Tel **01483 571 122**

| | |
|---|---|
| Mastectomies performed | 48 |
| Mastectomy wait in days | 18 |
| Lumpectomies performed | 5 |
| Lumpectomy wait in days | 19 |

*% of patients provided with*

| | |
|---|---|
| written information | 55% |
| support group information | 91% |

**Breast surgeons:**
Mark Kissin, Graham Layer (from November 2002)

**Patients referred to:**
Chemotherapy, radiotherapy, complex reconstruction, nuclear medicine, cancer genetics and Sentinel Node Mapping available on site

## St Peter's Hospital
Guildford Road, Chertsey, Surrey KT16 0PZ
Tel **01932 872 000**

| | |
|---|---|
| Mastectomies performed | 23 |
| Mastectomy wait in days | 20 |
| Lumpectomies performed | 21 |
| Lumpectomy wait in days | 22 |

*% of patients provided with*

| | |
|---|---|
| written information | 72% |
| support group information | 76% |

---

## Surrey BSU
Farnham Community Hospital
Hale Road, Farnham, Surrey GU9 9QL
Tel **01483 782 000**

Patients are currently screened within 35 months

| | | *98/9* | *99/0* | *00/1* |
|---|---|---|---|---|
| Pre-operative diagnosis rate 90% | | | | |
| Small cancer detection rate 3.1 | SDR | 1.20 | 1.22 | 1.32 |

---

# Sussex Cancer Network

### Royal Sussex County Hospital
Eastern Road, Brighton, East Sussex BN2 5BE
Tel 01273 696 955

| | |
|---|---|
| Mastectomies performed | 80 |
| Mastectomy wait in days | 35 |
| Lumpectomies performed | 55 |
| Lumpectomy wait in days | 28 |

*% of patients provided with*
| | |
|---|---|
| written information | 75% |
| support group information | 69% |

**Patients referred to:**
Sussex Cancer Centre for radiotherapy and chemotherapy

### Worthing Hospital
Lyndhurst Road, Worthing, West Sussex BN11 2DH
Tel 01903 205 111

| | |
|---|---|
| Mastectomies performed | 106 |
| Mastectomy wait in days | 11.5 |
| Lumpectomies performed | 161 |
| Lumpectomy wait in days | 9 |

*% of patients provided with*
| | |
|---|---|
| written information | 69% |
| support group information | 73% |

**Breast surgeons:**
Mr Asad Salman

---

### East Sussex BSU
Royal Sussex County Hospital
Eastern Road, Brighton, East Sussex BN2 5BE
Tel 01273 696 955

Patients are currently screened within 34-38 months

| | | | 98/9 | 99/0 | 00/1 |
|---|---|---|---|---|---|
| Pre-operative diagnosis rate | 88% | | | | |
| Small cancer detection rate | 3.0 | SDR | 1.06 | 1.32 | 1.06 |

### West Sussex BSU
Worthing Hospital
Lyndhurst Road, Worthing, West Sussex BN11 2DH
Tel 01903 205 111

Patients are currently screened within 34 months

| | | | 98/9 | 99/0 | 00/1 |
|---|---|---|---|---|---|
| Pre-operative diagnosis rate | 87% | | | | |
| Small cancer detection rate | 1.9 | SDR | 1.12 | 1.00 | 1.04 |

---

# Teeside, South Durham and North Yorkshire Cancer Network

## Bishop Auckland General Hospital
Cockton Hill Road, Bishop Auckland, County Durham DL14 6AD
Tel **01388 455 000**

| | |
|---|---|
| Mastectomies performed | 56 |
| Mastectomy wait in days | 17 |
| Lumpectomies performed | 30 |
| Lumpectomy wait in days | 18 |

*% of patients provided with*
| | |
|---|---|
| written information | 62% |
| support group information | 72% |

## Darlington Memorial Hospital
Hollyhurst Road, Darlington, County Durham DL3 6HX
Tel **01325 380 100**

| | |
|---|---|
| Mastectomies performed | 56 |
| Mastectomy wait in days | 17 |
| Lumpectomies performed | 30 |
| Lumpectomy wait in days | 18 |

*% of patients provided with*
| | |
|---|---|
| written information | 62% |
| support group information | 72% |

## Friarage Hospital
Northallerton, North Yorkshire DL6 1JG
Tel **01609 779 911**

| | |
|---|---|
| Mastectomies performed | 17 |
| Mastectomy wait in days | 18 |
| Lumpectomies performed | 10 |
| Lumpectomy wait in days | 14.5 |

*% of patients provided with*
| | |
|---|---|
| written information | 73% |
| support group information | 85% |

**Breast surgeons:**
Mr Robert Bryan, Mr M S Coady

**Patients referred to:**
James Cook University Hospital for radiotherapy and breast reconstruction

## University Hospital of Hartlepool

Holdforth Road, Hartlepool, Cleveland TS24 9AH
Tel **01429 266 654**

| | |
|---|---|
| Mastectomies performed | 80 |
| Mastectomy wait in days | 8 |
| Lumpectomies performed | 21 |
| Lumpectomy wait in days | 7 |

*% of patients provided with*
| | |
|---|---|
| written information | 66% |
| support group information | 69% |

## University Hospital of North Tees

Hardwick, Stockton-on-Tees, Cleveland TS19 8PE
Tel **01642 617 617**

| | |
|---|---|
| Mastectomies performed | 80 |
| Mastectomy wait in days | 8 |
| Lumpectomies performed | 21 |
| Lumpectomy wait in days | 7 |

*% of patients provided with*
| | |
|---|---|
| written information | 66% |
| support group information | 69% |

# Three Counties Cancer Network

## Cheltenham General Hospital
Sandford Road, Cheltenham, Gloucestershire GL53 7AN
Tel **01242 222 222**

| | |
|---|---|
| Mastectomies performed | 59 |
| Mastectomy wait in days | 14 |
| Lumpectomies performed | 28 |
| Lumpectomy wait in days | 14 |

*% of patients provided with*
| | |
|---|---|
| written information | 60% |
| support group information | 61% |

## County Hospital
Stonebow Road, Hereford HR1 2ER
Tel **01432 355 444**

| | |
|---|---|
| Mastectomies performed | 77 |
| Mastectomy wait in days | 7 |
| Lumpectomies performed | 25 |
| Lumpectomy wait in days | 7 |

*% of patients provided with*
| | |
|---|---|
| written information | 63% |
| support group information | 69% |

**Breast surgeons:**
Mr Allan Corder

**Patients referred to:**
Cheltenham General Hospital for radiotherapy
Wordsley Hospital for breast reconstruction

## Gloucestershire Royal Hospital
Great Western Road, Gloucester, Gloucestershire GL1 3NN
Tel **01452 528 555**

| | |
|---|---|
| Mastectomies performed | 33 |
| Mastectomy wait in days | 11 |
| Lumpectomies performed | 20 |
| Lumpectomy wait in days | 11.5 |

*% of patients provided with*
| | |
|---|---|
| written information | 61% |
| support group information | 69% |

## Stroud General Hospital
Trinity Road, Stroud, Gloucestershire GL5 2HY
Tel 01453 562 200

| | |
|---|---|
| Mastectomies performed | 7 |
| Mastectomy wait in days | 24 |
| Lumpectomies performed | 3 |
| Lumpectomy wait in days | 8 |

*% of patients provided with*
written information | -
support group information | -

## Worcester Royal Hospital
Ronkswood Branch, Newtown Road, Worcester WR5 1HN
Tel 01905 763 333

| | |
|---|---|
| Mastectomies performed | 149 |
| Mastectomy wait in days | 14 |
| Lumpectomies performed | 71 |
| Lumpectomy wait in days | 9 |

*% of patients provided with*
written information | 49%
support group information | 75%

---

## Gloucestershire BSU
Linton House, Cheltenham General Hospital
Thirlestaine Road, Cheltenham, Gloucestershire GL53 7AS
Tel 01242 222 222

Patients are currently screened within 36 months

| | | | 98/9 | 99/0 | 00/1 |
|---|---|---|---|---|---|
| Pre-operative diagnosis rate | 89% | | | | |
| Small cancer detection rate | 3.0 | SDR | 1.30 | 1.08 | 1.30 |

---

# West Anglia Cancer Network

## Addenbrooke's Hospital

Hills Road, Cambridge, Cambridgeshire CB2 2QQ
Tel **01223 245 151**

| | |
|---|---|
| Mastectomies performed | 97 |
| Mastectomy wait in days | 17.5 |
| Lumpectomies performed | 5 |
| Lumpectomy wait in days | 14 |

*% of patients provided with*
| | |
|---|---|
| written information | 73% |
| support group information | 76% |

**Breast surgeons:**
Mr A Purushotham

## Bedford Hospital

Kempston Road, Bedford MK42 9DJ
Tel **01234 355122**

| | |
|---|---|
| Mastectomies performed | 39 |
| Mastectomy wait in days | 13 |
| Lumpectomies performed | 14 |
| Lumpectomy wait in days | 12 |

*% of patients provided with*
| | |
|---|---|
| written information | 50% |
| support group information | 67% |

## Edith Cavell Hospital

Bretton Gate, Peterborough, Cambridgeshire PE3 9GZ
Tel **01733 874 000**

| | |
|---|---|
| Mastectomies performed | 75 |
| Mastectomy wait in days | 13 |
| Lumpectomies performed | 31 |
| Lumpectomy wait in days | 11 |

*% of patients provided with*
| | |
|---|---|
| written information | 77% |
| support group information | 81% |

**Patients referred to:**
Addenbrooke's Hospital (service starts 2002-2003)
Royal Marsden Hospital for breast reconstuction

## Hinchingbrooke Hospital

Hinchingbrooke Park, Huntingdon, Cambridgeshire PE29 6NT
Tel **01480 416 416**

| | |
|---|---|
| Mastectomies performed | 30 |
| Mastectomy wait in days | 0 |
| Lumpectomies performed | 4 |
| Lumpectomy wait in days | 0 |
| *% of patients provided with* | |
| written information | 64% |
| support group information | - |

**Breast surgeons:**
Mr John Benson, Mr Michael Urwin

## Princess Alexandra Hospital

Hamstel Road, Harlow, Essex CM20 1QX
Tel **01279 444 455**

| | |
|---|---|
| Mastectomies performed | 64 |
| Mastectomy wait in days | 15 |
| Lumpectomies performed | 12 |
| Lumpectomy wait in days | 17.5 |
| *% of patients provided with* | |
| written information | - |
| support group information | 73% |

## Queen Elizabeth Hospital

Gayton Road, King's Lynn, Norfolk PE30 4ET
Tel **01553 613 613**

| | |
|---|---|
| Mastectomies performed | 47 |
| Mastectomy wait in days | 12 |
| Lumpectomies performed | 15 |
| Lumpectomy wait in days | 15.5 |
| *% of patients provided with* | |
| written information | 69% |
| support group information | 78% |

**Breast surgeons:**
Mr Peter Gougu, Mr Surjait Singh

**Patients referred to:**
Addenbrooke's Hospital for oncology and radiotherapy
Norfolk and Norwich Hospital for plastic surgery and radiotherapy

## West Suffolk Hospital

Hardwick Lane, Bury St Edmunds, Suffolk IP33 2QZ
Tel 01284 713 000

| | |
|---|---|
| Mastectomies performed | 52 |
| Mastectomy wait in days | 14 |
| Lumpectomies performed | 7 |
| Lumpectomy wait in days | 11 |

*% of patients provided with*

| | |
|---|---|
| written information | 72% |
| support group information | 76% |

**Breast surgeons:**
Mr E Coveney, Mr O Ravisekar

**Patients referred to:**
Addenbrooke's Hospital for radiotherapy

---

## Cambridge and Huntingdon BSU

Addenbrookes Hospital
Hills Road, Cambridge, Cambridgeshire CB2 2QQ
Tel 01223 245 151

Currently, 95% of patients are screened within 36 months

| | | | 98/9 | 99/0 | 00/1 |
|---|---|---|---|---|---|
| Pre-operative diagnosis rate 85% | | | | | |
| Small cancer detection rate 3.7 | SDR | | 1.70 | 1.10 | 1.70 |

### Kings Lynn BSU

The Queen Elizabeth Hospital
Gayton Road, King's Lynn, Norfolk PE30 4ET
Tel 01553 613 613

Patients are currently screened within 38 months

| | | | 98/9 | 99/0 | 00/1 |
|---|---|---|---|---|---|
| Pre-operative diagnosis rate 90% | | | | | |
| Small cancer detection rate 2.5 | SDR | | 0.60 | 1.17 | 0.94 |

### West Essex and Redbridge BSU

St Margaret's Hospital
The Plain, Epping, Essex CM16 6TN
Tel 01279 444 455

Currently, 55% of patients are screened within 36 months

| | | | 98/9 | 99/0 | 00/1 |
|---|---|---|---|---|---|
| Pre-operative diagnosis rate 80% | | | | | |
| Small cancer detection rate 2.4 | SDR | | 1.04 | 1.04 | 1.22 |

## West Suffolk BSU

West Suffolk Hospital
Hardwick Lane, Bury St Edmunds, Suffolk IP33 2QZ
Tel 01284 713 000

Patients are currently screened within 38 months

| | | 98/9 | 99/0 | 00/1 |
|---|---|---|---|---|
| Pre-operative diagnosis rate 93% | | | | |
| Small cancer detection rate 3.5 | SDR | 1.09 | 1.03 | 1.15 |

# West London Cancer Network

## Central Middlesex Hospital
Acton Lane, Park Royal, London NW10 7NS
Tel **020 8965 5733**

| | |
|---|---|
| Mastectomies performed | 43 |
| Mastectomy wait in days | 16.5 |
| Lumpectomies performed | 7 |
| Lumpectomy wait in days | 21 |
| *% of patients provided with* | |
| written information | 52% |
| support group information | 71% |

## Charing Cross Hospital
Fulham Palace Road, Hammersmith, London W6 8RF
Tel **020 8383 0000**

| | |
|---|---|
| Mastectomies performed | 58 |
| Mastectomy wait in days | 6 |
| Lumpectomies performed | 41 |
| Lumpectomy wait in days | 8.5 |
| *% of patients provided with* | |
| written information | 45% |
| support group information | 64% |

## Chelsea and Westminster Hospital
369 Fulham Road, London SW10 9NH
Tel **020 8746 8000**

| | |
|---|---|
| Mastectomies performed | - |
| Mastectomy wait in days | - |
| Lumpectomies performed | - |
| Lumpectomy wait in days | - |
| *% of patients provided with* | |
| written information | - |
| support group information | - |

## Ealing Hospital
Uxbridge Road, Southall, Middlesex UB1 3HW
Tel **020 8967 5000**

| | |
|---|---|
| Mastectomies performed | 20 |
| Mastectomy wait in days | 11 |
| Lumpectomies performed | 10 |
| Lumpectomy wait in days | 5 |

*% of patients provided with*
written information          -
support group information    -

**Patients referred to:**
Charing Cross Hospital for radiotherapy, chemotherapy and breast
reconstruction

## Hillingdon Hospital
Pield Heath Road, Uxbridge, Middlesex UB8 3NN
Tel **01895 238 282**

| | |
|---|---|
| Mastectomies performed | 35 |
| Mastectomy wait in days | 15.5 |
| Lumpectomies performed | 15 |
| Lumpectomy wait in days | 16 |

*% of patients provided with*
written information          -
support group information    -

**Breast surgeons:**
Mr Addie Grobbelaar (based at Mount Vernon Hospital plastic surgery
unit), Mr Vahan Kaplan, Mr Christopher Kelley, Mr Brian Shoorey

**Patients referred to:**
Mount Vernon Hospital for oncology, adjuvant treatment, plastic
surgery and delayed or immediate breast reconstruction

## Northwick Park Hospital
Watford Road, Harrow, Middlesex HA1 3UJ
Tel **020 8864 3232**

| | |
|---|---|
| Mastectomies performed | 43 |
| Mastectomy wait in days | 16.5 |
| Lumpectomies performed | 7 |
| Lumpectomy wait in days | 21 |

*% of patients provided with*
written information       52%
support group information    71%

## St Mary's Hospital
Praed Street, Paddington, London W2 1NY
Tel **020 7886 6666**

| | |
|---|---|
| Mastectomies performed | 29 |
| Mastectomy wait in days | 8 |
| Lumpectomies performed | 4 |
| Lumpectomy wait in days | 8 |

*% of patients provided with*
written information        67%
support group information   82%

**Breast surgeons:**
Mr D Hadjiminas, Mr Simon Wood

# West Middlesex University Hospital
Twickenham Road, Isleworth, Middlesex TW7 6AF
Tel 020 8560 2121

| | |
|---|---|
| Mastectomies performed | 20 |
| Mastectomy wait in days | 7.5 |
| Lumpectomies performed | 10 |
| Lumpectomy wait in days | 12 |

*% of patients provided with*
written information       -
support group information   -

**Breast surgeons:**
Mr Rajev Vashisht

**Patients referred to:**
Charing Cross Hospital for radiotherapy and chemotherapy

---

# West of London BSU
Charing Cross Hospital
Fulham Palace Road, Hammersmith, London W6 8RF
Tel 020 8383 0000

Service did not operate for 7 months in 2001, so patients are currently screened within 42 months

| | | | 98/9 | 99/0 | 00/1 |
|---|---|---|---|---|---|
| Pre-operative diagnosis rate | 76% | | | | |
| Small cancer detection rate | 3.0 | SDR | 1.27 | 1.19 | 1.25 |

---

# Yorkshire Cancer Network

## Airedale General Hospital
Skipton Road, Steeton, West Yorkshire BD20 6TD
Tel **01535 652 511**

| | |
|---|---|
| Mastectomies performed | 26 |
| Mastectomy wait in days | 9 |
| Lumpectomies performed | 2 |
| Lumpectomy wait in days | 4 |

*% of patients provided with*
| | |
|---|---|
| written information | 57% |
| support group information | 76% |

## Bradford Royal Infirmary
Duckworth Lane, Bradford, West Yorkshire BD9 6RJ
Tel **01274 542 200**

| | |
|---|---|
| Mastectomies performed | 81 |
| Mastectomy wait in days | 26 |
| Lumpectomies performed | 22 |
| Lumpectomy wait in days | 28.5 |

*% of patients provided with*
| | |
|---|---|
| written information | 66% |
| support group information | 82% |

**Breast surgeons:**
Mr I T Fou, Professor Sharpe

**Patients referred to:**
Cookridge Hospital for radiotherapy

## Calderdale Royal Hospital
Huddersfield Road, Halifax, West Yorkshire HX3 0PW
Tel **01422 357 171**

| | |
|---|---|
| Mastectomies performed | 33 |
| Mastectomy wait in days | 6 |
| Lumpectomies performed | 3 |
| Lumpectomy wait in days | 2 |

*% of patients provided with*
| | |
|---|---|
| written information | 75% |
| support group information | 74% |

**Patients referred to:**
Bradford Royal Infirmary for breast reconstruction
Cookridge Hospital for radiotherapy
Huddersfield Royal Infirmary for chemotherapy

## Clayton Hospital

Northgate, Wakefield, Yorkshire, WF1 3JS
Tel 01924 201 688

Hospital also provides services for Pinderfields and Pontefract Hospitals

| | |
|---|---|
| Mastectomies performed | 84 |
| Mastectomy wait in days | 11 |
| Lumpectomies performed | 22 |
| Lumpectomy wait in days | 14 |

*% of patients provided with*
| | |
|---|---|
| written information | 44% |
| support group information | 80% |

**Breast surgeons:**
Mr Dedar Ali, Ms Orla Austen, Mr Craig Irvine, Mr Jit Parmar,
Mr Le Roux Fourie

**Patients referred to:**
Cookridge Hospital for radiotherapy

## Dewsbury and District Hospital

Halifax Road, Dewsbury, West Yorkshire WF13 4HS
Tel 01924 512 000

| | |
|---|---|
| Mastectomies performed | 36 |
| Mastectomy wait in days | 8 |
| Lumpectomies performed | 14 |
| Lumpectomy wait in days | 6 |

*% of patients provided with*
| | |
|---|---|
| written information | 58% |
| support group information | 85% |

## Harrogate District Hospital

Lancaster Park Road, Harrogate, North Yorkshire HG2 7SX
Tel 01423 885 959

| | |
|---|---|
| Mastectomies performed | 24 |
| Mastectomy wait in days | 16 |
| Lumpectomies performed | 5 |
| Lumpectomy wait in days | 13 |

*% of patients provided with*
| | |
|---|---|
| written information | - |
| support group information | - |

**Patients referred to:**
Cookridge Hospital for radiotherapy

## Huddersfield Royal Infirmary

Acre Street, Huddersfield, Yorkshire HD3 3EA
Tel 01484 342 000

| | |
|---|---|
| Mastectomies performed | 59 |
| Mastectomy wait in days | 17 |
| Lumpectomies performed | 4 |
| Lumpectomy wait in days | 4.5 |

*% of patients provided with*

| | |
|---|---|
| written information | 68% |
| support group information | 75% |

## Leeds General Infirmary

Great George Street, Leeds, West Yorkshire LS1 3EX
Tel 0113 243 2799

| | |
|---|---|
| Mastectomies performed | 175 |
| Mastectomy wait in days | 7 |
| Lumpectomies performed | 40 |
| Lumpectomy wait in days | 8 |

*% of patients provided with*

| | |
|---|---|
| written information | 47% |
| support group information | 74% |

**Breast surgeons:**
Miss M Bello, Mr K Horgan

**Patients referred to:**
Cookridge Hospital for radiotherapy and chemotherapy

## St James's University Hospital

Beckett Street, Leeds, West Yorkshire LS9 7TF
Tel 0113 243 3144

| | |
|---|---|
| Mastectomies performed | 175 |
| Mastectomy wait in days | 7 |
| Lumpectomies performed | 40 |
| Lumpectomy wait in days | 8 |

*% of patients provided with*

| | |
|---|---|
| written information | 47% |
| support group information | 74% |

**Patients referred to:**
Cookridge Hospital for radiotherapy

## York District Hospital

Wigginton Road, York, Yorkshire YO31 8HE
Tel 01904 631 313

| | |
|---|---|
| Mastectomies performed | 77 |
| Mastectomy wait in days | 19 |
| Lumpectomies performed | 20 |
| Lumpectomy wait in days | 18 |

*% of patients provided with*
written information 73%
support group information 75%

**Breast surgeons:**
Mr B Mancey-Jones, Mr S Nicholson

**Patients referred to:**
Cookridge Hospital for radiotherapy and chemotherapy

---

## Leeds and Wakefield BSU

Seacroft Hospital
York Road, Leeds, Yorkshire LS14 6UH
Tel 01132 648 164

Current screening interval not available

| | | | 98/9 | 99/0 | 00/1 |
|---|---|---|---|---|---|
| Pre-operative diagnosis rate 84% | | | | | |
| Small cancer detection rate 2.6 | SDR | | 1.22 | 1.21 | 1.24 |

## North Yorkshire BSU

York District Hospital
Wigginton Road, York, Yorkshire YO31 8HE
Tel 01904 631 313

Patients are currently screened within 34 months

| | | | 98/9 | 99/0 | 00/1 |
|---|---|---|---|---|---|
| Pre-operative diagnosis rate 95% | | | | | |
| Small cancer detection rate 2.7 | SDR | | 1.44 | 1.20 | 1.55 |

## Pennine BSU

Bradford Royal Infirmary
Duckworth Lane, Bradford, West Yorkshire BD9 6RJ
Tel 01274 542 200

Currently, 95% of patients are screened within 36 months

| | | | 98/9 | 99/0 | 00/1 |
|---|---|---|---|---|---|
| Pre-operative diagnosis rate - | | | | | |
| Small cancer detection rate - | SDR | | - | - | - |

# North and Mid Wales Cancer Network

**Glan Clwyd District General Hospital**
Bodelwyddan, Rhyl, Clwyd, Wales LL18 5UJ
Tel **01745 583 910**

**Wrexham Maelor Hospital**
Croesnewydd Road, Wrexham, Clwyd, Wales LL13 7TD
Tel **01978 291 100**

Breast surgeons:
Richard Cochrane, Jonathon Pye, Philip Richards

Patients referred to:
Glan Clwyd for radiotherapy

**Ysbyty Gwynedd**
Penrhosgarnedd, Bangor, Gwynedd, Wales LL57 2PW
Tel **01248 384 384**

# South East Wales Cancer Network

**Bronglais General Hospital**
Aberystwyth, Ceredigion, Dyfed, Wales SY23 1ER
Tel 01970 623 131

**Llandough Hospital**
Penlan Road, Llandough, Penarth, Vale of Glamorgan, Wales CF64 2XX
Tel 029 2071 1711

**Prince Charles Hospital**
Gurnos Estate, Merthyr Tydfil, Mid Glamorgan, Wales CF47 9DT
Tel 01685 721 721

**Royal Glamorgan Hospital**
Ynysmaerdy, Llantrisant, Mid Glamorgan, Wales CF72 8XR
Tel 01443 443 443

Breast surgeons:
Mr Eifion Vaughan-Williams, Mr Rhodri J L I Williams

Patients referred to:
Velindre Hospital for radiotherapy and chemotherapy

**Royal Gwent Hospital**
Cardiff Road, Newport, Gwent, Wales NP20 2UB
Tel 01633 234 234

Patients referred to:
Velindre Hospital for radiotherapy

**University Hospital of Wales**
Heath Park, Cardiff, Wales CF14 4XW
Tel 029 2074 7747

# South West Wales Cancer Network

**Prince Philip Hospital**
Bryngwynmawr, Llanelli, Wales SA14 8QF
Tel **01554 756 567**

**Patients referred to:**
Singleton Hospital for radiotherapy and chemotherapy

**Princess of Wales Hospital**
Coity Road, Bridgend, Glamorgan, Wales CF31 1RQ
Tel **01656 752 752**

**Singleton Hospital**
Sketty Road, Swansea, Wales SA2 8QA
Tel **01792 205 666**

**Breast surgeons:**
Mr M Chare-Morriston, Mr A Z Demian, Mr M C Mason

**Withybush General Hospital**
Fishguard Road, Haverfordwest, Pembrokeshire, Wales SA61 2PZ
Tel **01437 764 545**

**Breast surgeons:**
Mr Cooper, Mr M S Jafri, Mr W A Maxwell

**Patients referred to:**
Singleton Hospital for chemotherapy, radiotherapy and breast reconstruction

# North of Scotland Cancer Network

**Aberdeen Royal Infirmary**
Foresthill, Aberdeen, Scotland AB25 2ZN
Tel **01224 681 818**

# South East of Scotland Cancer Network

**Borders General Hospital**
Melrose, Roxburghshire, Scotland TD6 9BS
Tel **01896 826 000**

**Breast surgeons:**
Mr John S O'Neil

**Patients referred to:**
St John's Hospital at Howden for cosmetic and complex reconstructive surgery
Western General Hospital for radiotherapy and some chemotherapy

**Monklands Hospital**
Monkscourt Avenue, Airdrie, Lanarkshire, Scotland ML6 0JS
Tel **01236 748 748**

**Queen Margaret Hospital**
Whitefield Road, Dunfermline, Fife, Scotland KY12 0SU
Tel **01383 623 623**

**Patients referred to:**
Ninewells Hospital for radiotherapy and chemotherapy
Western General Hospital for radiotherapy and chemotherapy

---

**South East Scotland BSU**
Ardmillan House
42 Ardmillan Terrace, Edinburgh, Scotland EH11 2JL
Tel **0131 537 7410**

Patients are currently screened within 36 months

| | | 98/9 | 99/0 | 00/1 |
|---|---|---|---|---|
| Pre-operative diagnosis rate 83% | | | | |
| Small cancer detection rate 2.4 | SDR | 1.00 | 1.40 | - |

---

# West of Scotland Cancer Network

**Inverclyde Royal Hospital**
Larkfield Road, Greenock, Renfrewshire, Scotland PA16 0XN
Tel **01457 633 777**

**Breast surgeons:**
Mr J J Morrice, Mr E W Taylor

**Patients referred to:**
Beatson Oncology Centre for radiotherapy and inpatient chemotherapy
Canniesburn Hospital for breast reconstruction
Glasgow Homeopathic Hospital for homeopathy

# Northern Ireland

### Antrim Hospital
45 Bush Road, Antrim, County Antrim, N Ireland BT41 2RL
Tel **028 9442 4000**

### Causeway Hospital
Newbridge Road, Coleraine, County Londonderry, N Ireland BT52 1TT
Tel **028 7032 7032**

Causeway Hospital staff participate in multi-disciplinary team at Antrim
Hospital. Surgeon from Causeway Hospital conducts clinics and
diagnostic work in Antrim Hospital and performs surgery in Causeway
Hospital.

### Ulster Hospital
Upper Newtownards Road, Dundonald, Belfast, N Ireland BT16 0RH
Tel **028 9048 4511**

**Patients referred to:**
Belvoir Park Hospital for radiotherapy

---

### Northern Ireland Breast Screening Service
12-22 Linenhall Street, Belfast, N Ireland BT2 8BS
Tel **028 9033 3700**

Patients are currently screened within 38 months

| | | 98/9 | 99/0 | 00/1 |
|---|---|---|---|---|
| Pre-operative diagnosis rate 90% | | | | |
| Small cancer detection rate 2.6 | SDR | 0.94 | 1.20 | 1.24 |

---

# Five-year survival rates by HA

| Health Authority | Survival Rate[1] |
|---|---|
| England | 75.9 |
| Avon HA | 77.3 |
| Barking & Havering HA | 74.2 |
| Barnet, Enfield & Haringey HA | 75.3 |
| Barnsley HA | 72.2 |
| Bedfordshire HA | 77.7 |
| Berkshire HA | 76.9 |
| Bexley, Greenwich & Bromley HA | 81.3 |
| Birmingham HA | 78.0 |
| Bradford HA | 74.2 |
| Brent & Harrow HA | 77.6 |
| Buckinghamshire HA | 78.8 |
| Bury & Rochdale HA | 73.3 |
| Calderdale & Kirklees HA | 73.9 |
| Cambridgeshire HA | 78.7 |
| Camden & Islington HA | 79.8 |
| Cornwall & Isles of Scilly HA | 76.5 |
| County Durham & Darlington HA | 73.8 |
| Coventry HA | 76.8 |
| Croydon HA | 84.0 |
| Doncaster HA | 69.0 |
| Dorset HA | 71.8 |
| Dudley HA | 74.8 |
| Ealing, Hammersmith & Hounslow HA | 75.4 |
| East Kent HA | 79.4 |
| East Lancashire HA | 77.6 |
| East London & City HA | 66.7 |
| East Riding & Hull HA | 73.6 |
| East Surrey HA | 86.7 |
| East Sussex HA | 74.3 |
| Gateshead & South Tyneside HA | 73.8 |
| Gloucestershire HA | 75.6 |
| Herefordshire HA | 84.2 |
| Hertfordshire HA | 79.9 |
| Hillingdon HA | 78.0 |

| | |
|---|---|
| Isle of Wight, Portsmouth & SE Hampshire HA | 72.0 |
| Kensington, Chelsea & Westminster HA | 78.9 |
| Kingston & Richmond HA | 78.5 |
| Lambeth, Southwark & Lewisham HA | 74.1 |
| Leeds HA | 80.3 |
| Leicestershire HA | 76.7 |
| Lincolnshire HA | 72.2 |
| Liverpool HA | 69.8 |
| Manchester HA | 75.7 |
| Merton, Sutton & Wandsworth HA | 80.2 |
| Morecambe Bay HA | 73.5 |
| Newcastle & North Tyneside HA | 64.8 |
| Norfolk HA | 77.7 |
| North & East Devon HA | 74.2 |
| North & Mid Hampshire HA | 72.1 |
| North Cheshire HA | 74.1 |
| North Cumbria HA | 70.8 |
| North Derbyshire HA | 70.0 |
| North Essex HA | 80.6 |
| North Nottinghamshire HA | 75.3 |
| North Staffordshire HA | 69.6 |
| North West Lancashire HA | 74.5 |
| North Yorkshire HA | 78.6 |
| Northamptonshire HA | 75.4 |
| Northumberland HA | 67.6 |
| Nottingham HA | 76.0 |
| Oxfordshire HA | 81.0 |
| Redbridge & Waltham Forest HA | 77.2 |
| Rotherham HA | 76.0 |
| Salford & Trafford HA | 73.8 |
| Sandwell HA | 75.2 |
| Sefton HA | 76.5 |
| Sheffield HA | 72.4 |
| Shropshire HA | 77.4 |
| Solihull HA | 78.1 |
| Somerset HA | 77.6 |
| South and West Devon HA | 77.5 |
| South Cheshire HA | 76.2 |
| South Essex HA | 77.2 |
| South Humber HA | 71.4 |
| South Lancashire HA | 75.8 |

| | |
|---|---|
| South Staffordshire HA | 76.8 |
| Southampton & SW Hampshire HA | 71.0 |
| Southern Derbyshire HA | 77.5 |
| St Helens & Knowsley HA | 76.2 |
| Stockport HA | 74.2 |
| Suffolk HA | 77.7 |
| Sunderland HA | 69.7 |
| Tees HA | 69.3 |
| Wakefield HA | 78.9 |
| Walsall HA | 73.1 |
| Warwickshire HA | 78.0 |
| West Kent HA | 78.4 |
| West Pennine HA | 71.8 |
| West Surrey HA | 78.4 |
| West Sussex HA | 77.9 |
| Wigan & Bolton HA | 77.0 |
| Wiltshire HA | 71.1 |
| Wirral HA | 74.3 |
| Wolverhampton HA | 74.6 |
| Worcestershire HA | 80.1 |

| Health Board[2] | Survival Rate[3] |
|---|---|
| **Scotland** | **73.2** |
| Argyll & Clyde | 72.8 |
| Airshire & Arran | 72.3 |
| Borders | 73.5 |
| Dumfries & Galloway | 73.4 |
| Fife | 74.9 |
| Forth Valley | 74.7 |
| Grampian | 75.1 |
| Greater Glasgow | 71.3 |
| Highland | 74.5 |
| Lanarkshire | 72.4 |
| Lothian | 74.1 |
| Tayside | 72.6 |

[1] Survival rate of patients first diagnosed 1993–95.
[2] Mainland Health Boards only. Figures for Scotland include Orkney, Shetland and Western Isles.
[3] Unadjusted survival rate of patients first diagnosed 1991–95. Cases diagnosed in 1994–95 do not have five years follow-up.
Source: NHS Performance Indicators 2002 and NHS Scotland National Statistics release.

# Private hospitals

The following private hospitals offer core cancer services *and* have a BUPA approved breast unit (see p.148):

**Ashtead • Ashtead Hospital**
☑ ☺ ⦿
The Warren, Ashtead
Surrey KT21 2SB
Tel 01372 276 161
Capio Healthcare Ltd
Insurers: BUPA*, PPP*, Norwich*, Standard
Life*, Royal Sun Alliance*, WPA

**Basingstoke • BMI The Hampshire Clinic**
☑ ☺
Basing Road, Old Basing, Basingstoke
Hampshire RG24 7AL
Tel 01256 357 111
General Healthcare Group Ltd
Insurers: BUPA*, PPP*, Norwich*, Standard
Life, Royal Sun Alliance*, WPA

**Bath • BMI Bath Clinic**
☑ ☺ ⦿
Claverton Down Road, Combe Down
Bath, Avon BA2 7BR
Tel 01225 835 555
General Healthcare Group
Insurers: BUPA*, PPP*, Norwich*, Standard
Life*, Royal Sun Alliance*, WPA

**Bingley • The Yorkshire Clinic**
☑ ☺
Bradford Road, Bingley
West Yorkshire BD16 1TW
Tel 01274 560 311
Capio Healthcare Ltd
Insurers: BUPA*, Norwich*, Standard Life*,
Royal Sun Alliance, WPA

**Birmingham • Birmingham Nuffield Hospital**
☑ ☺
22 Somerset Road, Edgbaston
Birmingham B15 2QQ
Tel 0121 456 2000
Nuffield Hospitals
Insurers: BUPA*, PPP, Norwich*, Standard
Life, Royal Sun Alliance*, WPA

**Birmingham • BMI The Priory Hospital**
☑ ☺ ⦿
Priory Rd, Edgbaston
Birmingham B5 7UG
Tel 0121 440 2323
General Healthcare Group
Insurers: BUPA*, PPP*, Norwich, Standard
Life, Royal Sun Alliance, WPA

**Blackburn • BMI The Beardwood Hospital**
☑
Preston New Road, Blackburn
Lancashire BB2 7AE
Tel 01254 507 607
General Healthcare Group
Insurers: BUPA*, PPP*, Norwich*, Standard
Life, Royal Sun Alliance*, WPA

**Brentwood • BUPA Hartswood Hospital**
☑ ☺ ⦿
Eagle Way, Brentwood
Essex CM13 3LE
Tel 01277 232 525
BUPA Hospitals
Insurers: BUPA, PPP, Norwich, Standard
Life, Royal Sun Alliance, WPA

**Bristol • Bristol Nuffield Hospital**
☑ ☺
Upper Byron Place, 3 Clifton Hill
Clifton, Bristol BS8 1BP
Tel 0117 973 0391
Nuffield Nursing Homes Trust
Insurers: BUPA*, Norwich*, Standard Life*,
Royal Sun Alliance*, WPA

**Cambridge • BUPA Cambridge Lea Hospital**
☑.
30 New Road, Impington
Cambridge CB4 9EL
Tel 01223 266 900
BUPA Hospitals
Insurers: BUPA, PPP, Norwich, Standard
Life, Royal Sun Alliance, WPA

**Cambridge • The Evelyn Hospital**
☑
4 Trumpington Road
Cambridge CB2 2AF
Tel 01223 303 336
Insurers: BUPA*, WPA

**Cheadle · BMI The Alexandra Hospital**
Mill Lane, Cheadle
Cheshire SK8 2PX
Tel 0161 428 3656
General Healthcare Group
Insurers: BUPA*, PPP*, Norwich*, Standard Life, Royal Sun Alliance*, WPA

**Chelmsford · Springfield Hospital**
Lawn Lane, Springfield
Chelmsford, Essex CM1 7GU
Tel 01245 234 000
Capio Healthcare Ltd
Insurers: BUPA*, PPP*, Norwich*, Standard Life*, Royal Sun Alliance*, WPA

**Chelsea · The Lister Hospital**
Chelsea Bridge Road
London SW1W 8RH
Tel 020 7730 3417
HCA International Ltd
Insurers: BUPA, PPP, Norwich, Standard Life, Royal Sun Alliance, WPA

**Cheltenham · Cheltenham General Hospital**
Sanford Road
Cheltenham GL53 7AN
Tel 01242 222 222
Insurers: WPA

**Chorley · Euxton Hall Hospital**
Wigan Road, Euxton, Chorley
Lancashire PR7 6DY
Tel 01257 276 261
Capio Healthcare Ltd
Insurers: BUPA*, PPP*, Norwich*, Standard Life*, Royal Sun Alliance*, WPA

**Colchester · The Oaks Hospital**
Oaks Place, Mile End Road, Colchester
Essex CO4 5XR
Tel 01206 752 121
Insurers: BUPA*, PPP*, Norwich*, Standard Life*, Royal Sun Alliance*, WPA

**Cottingham · Hull Nuffield Hospital**
Castle Hill Hospital, Castle Road
Cottingham, East Yorkshire HU16 5FQ
Tel 01482 623 500
Nuffield Hospitals
Insurers: BUPA*, Norwich, Standard Life, Royal Sun Alliance, WPA

**Croydon · BMI Shirley Oaks Hospital**
Poppy Lane, Shirley Oaks Village
Croydon, Surrey CR9 8AB
Tel 0208 655 5500
General Healthcare Group Ltd
Insurers: BUPA*, PPP, Norwich, Standard Life, WPA

**Derby · East Midlands Nuffield Hospital**
Rykneld Road, Littleover, Derby
Derbyshire DE23 7SN
Tel 01332 517 891
Insurers: BUPA*, PPP*, Norwich*, Standard Life*, Royal Sun Alliance*, WPA

**Eastleigh · Wessex Nuffield Hospital**
Winchester Road, Chandler's Ford
Eastleigh, Hampshire SO53 2DW
Tel 02380 266 377
Nuffield Hospitals
Insurers: BUPA*, PPP, Norwich*, Standard Life*, Royal Sun Alliance*, WPA

**Elland · BUPA Hospital Elland**
Elland Lane, Elland
West Yorkshire HX5 9EB
Tel 01422 324 000
BUPA Hospitals
Insurers: BUPA, PPP, Norwich, Standard Life, Royal Sun Alliance, WPA

**Enfield · North London Nuffield Hospital**
Cavell Drive, Uplands Park Road
Enfield, Middlesex EN2 7PR
Tel 020 8366 2122
Nuffield Nursing Homes Trust
Insurers: BUPA*, PPP, Norwich*, Standard Life*, Royal Sun Alliance*, WPA

**Enfield · BMI The King's Oak Hospital**
Chase Farm (North Side), The Ridgeway
Enfield, Middlesex EN2 8SD
Tel 020 8370 9500
General Healthcare Group Ltd
Insurers: BUPA*, PPP*, Norwich*, Royal Sun Alliance*, WPA

**Exeter • Exeter Nuffield Hospital**

✓ ✦

Wonford Road, Exeter
Devon EX2 4UG
**Tel 01392 276 591**
Nuffield Hospitals
Insurers: BUPA*, PPP, Norwich, Standard
Life, WPA

**Great Missenden • BMI The Chiltern Hospital**

✓ ✦

London Road, Great Missenden
Buckinghamshire HP16 0EN
**Tel 01494 890 890**
General Healthcare Group
Insurers: BUPA*, PPP*, Norwich*, Standard
Life, Royal Sun Alliance*, WPA

**Harpenden • BUPA Hospital Harpenden**

✓ ✦ ◑

Ambrose Lane, Harpenden
Herts AL5 4BP
**Tel 01582 763 191**
BUPA Hospitals
Insurers: BUPA, PPP, Norwich, Standard
Life, Royal Sun Alliance, WPA

**Harrow • Northwick Park Hospital**

✓

Watford Road, Harrow
Middlesex HA1 3UJ
**Tel 020 8864 3232**
Insurers: WPA

**Hythe • BUPA St Saviour's Hospital**

✓ ✦ ◑

73 Seabrook Road, Hythe
Kent CT21 5BU
**Tel 01303 265 581**
BUPA Hospitals
Insurers: BUPA, PPP, Norwich, Standard
Life, Royal Sun Alliance, WPA

**Ipswich • Suffolk Nuffield at Christchurch Park Hospital**

✓ ✦

57 Fonnereau Road, Ipswich
Suffolk IP1 3JN
**Tel 01473 256 071**
Insurers: BUPA*, PPP*, Norwich, Standard
Life, Royal Sun Alliance, WPA

**Ipswich • The Suffolk Nuffield at Foxhall**

✓ ✦

Foxhall Road, Ipswich
Suffolk IP4 5SW
**Tel 01473 279 100**
Insurers: BUPA*, PPP*, Norwich, Standard
Life, Royal Sun Alliance, WPA

**Kingston upon Thames • New Victoria Hospital**

✓ ✦

184 Coombe Lane West
Kingston upon Thames, Surrey KT2 7EG
**Tel 020 8949 9000**
Charitable Trust
Insurers: BUPA*, PPP*, Norwich, Standard
Life*, Royal Sun Alliance*, WPA

**Leamington Spa • Warwickshire Nuffield Hospital**

✓ ✦ ◑

The Chase, Leamington Spa
Warwickshire CV32 6RW
**Tel 01926 427 971**
Nuffield Hospitals
Insurers: BUPA*, PPP*, Norwich*, Standard
Life*, Royal Sun Alliance*, WPA

**Leicester • BUPA Hospital Leicester**

✓ ✦ ◑

Gartree Road, Oadby
Leicester LE2 2FF
**Tel 0116 272 0888**
BUPA Hospitals
Insurers: BUPA, PPP, Norwich, Standard
Life, Royal Sun Alliance, WPA

**London • Cromwell Hospital**

✓ ✦ ◑

Cromwell Road
London SW5 0TU
**Tel 020 7460 2000**
Insurers: PPP, Norwich, Standard Life,
Royal Sun Alliance, WPA

**London • Hospital of St John and St Elizabeth**

✓

60 Grove End Road, St John's Wood
London NW8 9NH
**Tel 020 7806 4000**
Insurers: BUPA*, WPA

**London • Royal Marsden Hospital**

✓

Fulham Road
London SW3 6JJ
**Tel 020 7352 8171**
Insurers: WPA

**Manchester · BUPA Hospital Manchester**

⊘ ✦

Russell Road, Whalley Range
Manchester M16 8AJ
**Tel 0161 226 0112**
BUPA Hospitals
Insurers: BUPA, PPP, Norwich, Standard
Life, Royal Sun Alliance, WPA

**Milton Keynes · BMI Saxon Clinic**

⊘ ✦ ①

Chadwick Drive, Saxon Street
Milton Keynes, Bucks MK6 5LR
**Tel 01908 665 533**
General Healthcare Group
Insurers: BUPA*, PPP*, Norwich*, Standard
Life, Royal Sun Alliance, WPA

**Newcastle upon Tyne · Newcastle Nuffield Hospital**

⊘ ✦ ①

Clayton Road, Jesmond
Newcastle upon Tyne NE2 1JP
**Tel 0191 281 6131**
Nuffield Nursing Homes Trust
Insurers: BUPA*, PPP*, Norwich*, Standard
Life*, Royal Sun Alliance*, WPA

**Northampton · BMI Three Shires Hospital**

⊘ ✦ ①

The Avenue, Cliftonville
Northampton NN1 5DR
**Tel 01604 620 311**
General Healthcare Group Ltd
Insurers: BUPA*, PPP*, Norwich*, Standard
Life*, Royal Sun Alliance*, WPA

**Northwood · BMI Bishops Wood Hospital**

⊘ ✦ ✦ ①

Rickmanworth Road, Northwood
Middlesex HA6 2JW
**Tel 01923 835 814**
General Healthcare Group
Insurers: BUPA*, PPP*, Norwich*, Royal
Sun Alliance*, WPA

**Nottingham · BMI The Park Hospital**

⊘ ✦ ①

Sherwood Lodge Drive, Arnold
Nottingham NG5 8RX
**Tel 0115 967 0670**
General Healthcare Group
Insurers: BUPA*, PPP*, Norwich*, Standard
Life*, Royal Sun Alliance*, WPA

**Oxford · The Acland Hospital**

⊘ ✦ ①

Banbury Road, Oxford
Oxfordshire OX2 6PD
**Tel 01865 404 142**
Nuffield Nursing Homes Trust
Insurers: BUPA*, PPP*, Norwich*, Standard
Life, Royal Sun Alliance, WPA

**Preston · Fulwood Hall Hospital**

⊘ ✦ ①

Midgery Lane, Fulwood, Preston
Lancashire PR2 9SZ
**Tel 01772 704 111**
Capio Healthcare Ltd
Insurers: BUPA*, PPP*, Norwich*, Standard
Life*, Royal Sun Alliance*, WPA

**Sawbridgeworth · Rivers Hospital**

⊘ ✦

High Wych Road, Sawbridgeworth
Hertfordshire CM21 0HH
**Tel 01279 600 282**
Capio Healthcare Ltd
Insurers: BUPA*, PPP*, Norwich*, Standard
Life*, Royal Sun Alliance*, WPA

**Shrewsbury · Shropshire Nuffield Hospital**

⊘

Longden Road, Shrewsbury
Shropshire SY3 9DP
**Tel 01743 282 500**
Nuffield Hospitals
Insurers: BUPA*, PPP*, Norwich*, Standard
Life*, Royal Sun Alliance*, WPA

**Slough · Thames Valley Nuffield Hospital**

⊘ ✦ ①

Wexham Sreet, Wexham, Slough
Berkshire SL3 6NH
**Tel 01753 662 241**
Nuffield Nursing Homes Trust
Insurers: BUPA, PPP, Norwich*, Standard
Life, Royal Sun Alliance, WPA

**Southend on Sea · BUPA Wellesley Hospital**

⊘ ✦ ①

Eastern Avenue, Southend on Sea
Essex SS2 4XH
**Tel 01702 462 944**
BUPA Hospitals
Insurers: BUPA, PPP, Norwich*, Standard
Life, Royal Sun Alliance, WPA

**Stafford · Rowley Hall Hospital**

Rowley Park
Stafford ST17 9DQ
**Tel 01785 223 203**
Community Hospitals Group
Insurers: BUPA*, PPP*, Norwich*, Standard
Life*, Royal Sun Alliance*, WPA

**Sutton Coldfield · BUPA Hospital
Little Aston**

Little Aston Hall Drive, Sutton
Coldfield, West Midlands B74 3UP
**Tel 0121 353 2444**
BUPA Hospitals
Insurers: BUPA, PPP, Norwich, Standard
Life, Royal Sun Alliance, WPA

**Swindon · BMI The Ridgeway
Hospital**

Moormead Road, Wroughton, Swindon
Wiltshire SN4 9DD
**Tel 01793 814 848**
General Healthcare Group Ltd
Insurers: BUPA*, PPP*, Norwich*, Standard
Life, Royal Sun Alliance, WPA

**Telford · Princess Royal Hospital**

Apley Castle
Telford TF1 6TF
**Tel 01952 641 222**
Insurers: WPA

**Tettenhall · Wolverhampton
Nuffield Hospital**

Wood Road, Tettenhall
Wolverhampton WV6 8LE
**Tel 01902 754 177**
Nuffield Nursing Homes Trust
Insurers: BUPA*, PPP*, Norwich*, Standard
Life*, Royal Sun Alliance*, WPA

**Walderslade · BUPA Alexandra
Hospital**

Impton Lane, Walderslade
Kent ME5 9PG
**Tel 01634 687 166**
BUPA Hospitals
Insurers: BUPA, PPP, Norwich, Standard
Life, WPA

**Warrington · BUPA North Cheshire
Hospital**

Fir Tree Close, Stretton, Warrington
Cheshire WA4 4LU
**Tel 01925 265000**
BUPA Hospitals
Insurers: BUPA, PPP, Norwich, Standard
Life, Royal Sun Alliance, WPA

**Windsor · BMI The Princess
Margaret Hospital**

Osborne Rd, Windsor
Berkshire SL4 3SJ
**Tel 01753 743 434**
General Healthcare Group
Insurers: BUPA*, PPP*, Norwich*, Standard
Life, Royal Sun Alliance*, WPA

**Windsor · HRH Princess Christian's
Hospital**

12 Clarence Road, Windsor
Berkshire SL4 5AG
**Tel 01753 853 121**
Nuffield Nursing Homes Trust
Insurers: BUPA*, Norwich*, Standard Life*,
Royal Sun Alliance*, WPA

**SCOTLAND**

**Edinburgh · BUPA Murrayfield
Hospital**

122 Corstorphine Road
Edinburgh EH12 6UD
**Tel 0131 334 0363**
BUPA Hospitals
Insurers: BUPA, PPP, Norwich*, Standard
Life, Royal Sun Alliance, WPA

The following private hospitals offer breast surgery and may have core cancer services, but *do not* have a BUPA approved breast unit:

**Barrow in Furness • Abbey Park Hospital**
Dalton Lane, Barrow in Furness
Cumbria LA14 4TP
Tel 01229 813 388
Insurers: BUPA*, PPP, Standard Life, WPA

**Blackpool • BUPA Fylde Coast Hospital**
St Walburgas Road, Blackpool
Lancashire FY3 8BP
Tel 01253 394 188
Insurers: BUPA, PPP, Norwich*, Standard Life, Royal Sun Alliance, WPA

**Carlisle • Abbey Caldew Hospital**
64 Dalston Road, Carlisle
Cumbria CA2 5NW
Tel 01228 531 713
Insurers: BUPA, PPP, Norwich, Standard Life, Royal Sun Alliance, WPA

**Chesterfield • BMI Chatsworth Suite**
Chesterfield Royal Hospital, Calow
Chesterfield, Derbyshire S44 5BL
Tel 01246 544 400
Insurers: BUPA*, PPP*, Norwich*, Standard Life, Royal Sun Alliance*, WPA

**Eastbourne • BMI Esperance Private Hospital**
Hartington Place, Eastbourne
East Sussex BN21 3BG
Tel 01323 411 188
Insurers: BUPA*, PPP*, Norwich, Royal Sun Alliance, WPA

**Farnham • BUPA Hospital Clare Park**
Clare Park, Crondale Lane
Farnham Surrey GU10 5XX
Tel 01252 850 216
Insurers: BUPA, PPP, Norwich, Standard Life, Royal Sun Alliance, WPA

**Guildford • Guildford Nuffield Hospital**
Stirling Road, Guildford
Surrey GU2 7RF
Tel 01483 555 800
Insurers: BUPA*, PPP*, Norwich*, Standard Life*, Royal Sun Alliance*, WPA

**Harrogate • Duchy Nuffield Hospital**
Queen's Road, Harrogate
North Yorkshire HG2 0HF
Tel 01423 567 136
Insurers: BUPA, PPP, Norwich*, Standard Life, Royal Sun Alliance, WPA

**Haywards Heath • Ashdown Nuffield Hospital**
The Burrell Road, Haywards Heath
West Sussex RH16 1UD
Tel 01444 456 999
Insurers: PPP, BUPA, Norwich*, Standard Life, WPA

**High Wycombe • BMI The Shelburne Hospital**
Queen Alexandra Road, High Wycombe
Buckinghamshire HP11 2TR
Tel 01494 888 700
Insurers: BUPA, PPP, Norwich*, Standard Life, Royal Sun Alliance*, WPA

**Hitchin • Pinehill Hospital**
Benslow Lane, Hitchin
Hertfordshire SG4 9QZ
Tel 01462 422 822
Insurers: BUPA*, PPP, Norwich*, Standard Life*, Royal Sun Alliance, WPA

**Leicester • Leicester Nuffield Hospital**
Scraptoft Lane, Leicester
Leicestershire LE5 1HY
Tel 0116 276 9401
Insurers: BUPA*, PPP, Norwich*, Standard Life*, Royal Sun Alliance*, WPA

**London • The London Clinic**
20 Devonshire Place
London W1G 6BW
Tel 020 7935 4444
Insurers: BUPA*, PPP*, Norwich, Royal Sun Alliance*, WPA

**Nottingham • The Nottingham Nuffield Hospital**
748 Mansfield Road, Woodthorpe
Nottingham, Nottinghamshire NG5 3FZ
Tel 0115 920 9209
Insurers: Norwich*, Standard Life, Royal
Sun Alliance, WPA

**Nuneaton • BMI Nuneaton Private Hospital**
132 Coventry Road, Nuneaton
Warwickshire CV10 7AD
Tel 02476 357 500
Insurers: BUPA*, PPP*, Norwich*, Standard
Life*, Royal Sun Alliance*, WPA

**Reading • Berkshire Independent Hospital**
⓪
Wensley Road, Coley Park
Reading, Surrey RG1 6UZ
Tel 0118 902 8000
Insurers: BUPA, PPP*, Norwich*, Standard
Life, Royal Sun Alliance, WPA

**Reading • BUPA Dunedin Hospital**
⊕ ⓪
16 Bath Road, Reading
Berkshire RG1 6NB
Tel 01189 587 676
Insurers: PPP, Norwich, Standard Life,
Royal Sun Alliance, WPA

**Redhill • BUPA Redwood Hospital**
⊕ ⓪
Canada Drive, Redhill
Surrey RH1 5BY
Tel 01737 277 277
Insurers: BUPA, PPP, Norwich, Standard
Life, Royal Sun Alliance, WPA

**St Leonards-on-Sea • BUPA Hospital Hastings**
⊕ ⓪
The Ridge, St Leonards-on-Sea
East Sussex TN37 7RE
Tel 01424 757 400
Insurers: BUPA, PPP, Norwich, Standard
Life, Royal Sun Alliance, WPA

**Stockton-on-Tees • Cleveland Nuffield Hospital**
⊕
Junction Road, Norton
Stockton-on-Tees, Cleveland TS20 1PX
Tel 01642 360 100
Insurers: BUPA*, PPP*, Norwich*, Standard
Life*, Royal Sun Alliance*, WPA

**Torquay • Mount Stuart Hospital**
St Vincents Road, Torquay
Devon TQ1 4UP
Tel 01803 313 881
Insurers: BUPA*, PPP*, Norwich*, Standard
Life, Royal Sun Alliance, WPA

**Winchester • BMI Sarum Road Hospital**
⊕ ⓪
Sarum Road, Winchester
Hampshire SO22 5HA
Tel 01962 844 555
Insurers: BUPA, PPP*, Norwich*, Standard
Life, Royal Sun Alliance, WPA

**Wrexham • BUPA Yale Hospital**
⊘
Wrexham Technology Park,
Croesnewydd Road
Wrexham, Wales LL13 7YP
Tel 01978 291 306
Insurers: BUPA, PPP, Norwich, Standard
Life, Royal Sun Alliance, WPA

# Methodology

The Dr Foster Guide to Breast Cancer was developed in consultation with UK Breast Cancer Care, Macmillan Cancer Relief, UK Breast Cancer Coalition, BASO, leading doctors (see page vi), the Department of Health and the UK NHS Breast Screening Service. The consultation identified a number of key issues in relation to hospital care for people with breast cancer. Data relating to these issues was addressed in a questionnaire to all symptomatic clinics and screening units in the UK. The questionnaires were circulated and completed in July/August 2002. Data definitions for screening units are as used for the KC62 screening service returns. The exception is the screening interval figure. In some cases units were not able to supply a figure for the current screening interval but were able to indicate the time taken to screen a set target percentage of patients. In these cases the alternative figure has been given.

The figures for the number of procedures performed and the waiting times for procedures for English units are derived from Hospital Episode Statistics for the year to March 2001. Hospital Episode Statistics include records of all inpatient episodes in UK hospitals including details of diagnosis and procedures performed. The figures relate to procedures performed on patients with a primary diagnosis of breast cancer.

# Useful addresses

**AICR**
The Association for International
Cancer Research
Aims to support research into the
causes, mechanisms, diagnosis,
treatment and prevention of cancer.
Madras House, South Street
St Andrews KY16 9EH
Tel 01334 477910
www.aicr.org.uk

**Breakthrough Breast Cancer**
Kingsway House, 103 Kingsway
London WC2B 6QX
Tel 020 7405 5111
www.breakthrough.org.uk
Email: info@breakthrough.org.uk

**Breast Cancer Care**
Kiln House, 210 New Kings Road
London SW6 4NZ
Tel 020 7384 2984
Freephone helpline
0808 800 6000
www.breastcancercare.org.uk
Email: info@breastcancercare.org.uk

**The Bristol Cancer Help Centre**
Offers healing and positive healthcare
to people affected by cancer, and to
their supporters.
Grove House, Cornwallis Grove
Bristol BS8 4PG
Tel 0117 980 9500
www.bristolcancerhelp.org

**CancerBACUP**
3 Bath Place, Rivington Street
London EC2A 3JR.
Freephone helpline
0808 800 1234
Tel 020 7739 2280
www.cancerbacup.org.uk

**Cancer Research UK**
P.O. Box 123
Lincoln's Inn Fields
London WC2A 3PX
Tel 020 7242 0200
www.cancerresearchuk.org

**Eloise Lingerie**
Provide a wide range of
mastectomy bras and swimwear.
PO Box 70, Bury St Edmunds
Suffolk IP 30 OJT
Tel 01284 828787
www.eloise.co.uk

**The Haven Trust**
A national charity dedicated to
providing a network of support centres.
Helpline 08707 272 273
www.thehaventrust.org.uk

**Lymphoedema Support Network**
St. Luke's Crypt, Sydney Street
London SW3 6NH
Tel 020 7351 0990
www.lymphoedema.org/lsn

**Macmillan Cancer Relief**
89 Albert Embankment
London SE1 7YQ
Macmillan Cancer Line:
Freephone helpline
0808 808 2020
www.macmillan.org.uk
Email: cancerline@macmillan.org.uk.

**Marie Curie Cancer Care**
89 Albert Embankment
London SE1 7TP
Tel 020 7599 7777
www.mariecurie.org.uk
Email: info@mariecurie.org.uk
Email: hospices@mariecurie.org.uk
Email: nursing@mariecurie.org.uk

## NHS Direct Online Breast Cancer Information
Tel 0845 4647
www.minervation.com/cancer/breast/patient

## PAC
Positive Action on Cancer
Free counselling service for those affected by breast and other cancers.
2a Market Place, Frome
Somerset BA11 1AG
Tel 01373 455 255
www.pacproject.co.uk
Email: info@pacproject.co.uk

## Tenovus
Funds support and counselling services for cancer patients and their families.
Velindre Hospital, Whitchurch
Cardiff CF14 2TL
Freephone helpline
0808 808 1010
www.tenovus.com/
Email: tcic@velindre-tr.wales.nhs.uk

## UKBCC
The UK Breast Cancer Coalition
Suite 1D, Broadway House
112–134 The Broadway
Wimbledon SW19 1RL
Tel 020 8543 4455
www.ukbcc.org.uk
Email: info@ukbcc.org.uk

## Dr Foster Help at Hand Service
Tel 0906 190 0212
www.drfoster.co.uk

## British Homeopathic Association & the Faculty of Homeopathy
Faculty members are medically trained healthcare professionals such as GPs.
Tel 020 7566 7800 (BHA)/
7810 (Faculty)
www.trusthomeopathy.org

## Society of Homeopaths
Society members have completed homeopathic degree but may have no other healthcare training.
Tel 01604 621400
www.homeopathy-soh.org

## The British Acupuncture Council
Members have over 1200 hours of training and abide by code of practice.
Tel 020 8735 0400
www.acupuncture.org.uk

## British Medical Acupuncture Society
Members practice acupuncture within the scope of their medical training.
Tel 01925 730727
www.medical-acupuncture.co.uk

## The Acupuncture Association of Chartered Physiotherapists
Members practice acupuncture within the scope of their medical training.
Tel 01747 861151
www.aacp.uk.com

## British Hypnotherapy Association
Sets standards in training and practice.
Tel 020 7723 4443

## The Register of Chinese Herbal Medicine
Members are qualified in Chinese medicine after studying for up to 4 yrs.
Tel 01603 623994
www.rchm.co.uk

## Members of these Western herbalist professional bodies are trained to a minimum of degree level:

## The National Institute of Medical Herbalists
Tel 01392 426022
www.nimh.org.uk

## Association of Master Herbalists
Tel 01482 887352

## The International Register of Consultant Herbalists
Tel 01792 655886
www.irch.org

# Glossary

**Abdominal hernia** A hernia protruding through a defect or weakened portion of the abdominal wall.

**Adjuvant treatment/therapy** Treatment given in addition to a primary therapy. For breast cancer, adjuvant treatment is usually chemotherapy, hormone treatment or radiotherapy given after surgery.

**Anastrozole** An aromatase inhibitor that reduces the amount of oestrogen in the body which many breast cancers rely on to grow.

**Areola** The circular field of dark-coloured skin surrounding the nipple.

**Aromatase inhibitors** Drugs that block the production of oestrogen by the adrenal glands and in fatty tissue. They are often used to treat breast cancer that has spread or metastasised.

**Atypical hyperplasia** Overgrowth of the breast cells.

**Axillary lymph nodes** A group of glands situated in the armpit.

**Axillary lymph node sampling/dissection** The removal of at least four axillary nodes to check whether the cancer has spread.

**Axillary node clearance** Surgical removal of the lymph nodes from the armpit.

**Benign** This term refers to a growth that is non-cancerous.

**Biological therapies** Therapies that harness the body's immune system to fight cancer.

**Biopsy** The removal of a sample of cells which are then examined under a microscope to check for abnormalities.

**Bone scan** A dose of a mild radioactive agent is injected into a vein and a scan reads the distribution of the radioactivity. More radioactivity is absorbed by areas of the bone affected by cancer.

**BRCA1** Women who carry this faulty gene have a higher chance of developing breast cancer than women who do not. It is associated with up to five out of 10 cases of inherited breast cancer in the UK.

**BRCA2** Women who carry this faulty gene have a higher chance of developing breast cancer than women who do not. It is associated with four out of 10 cases of inherited breast cancer in the UK.

**Breast** The adult female breast is composed of four structures:
1. Lobules/glands – glands are grouped in sections called lobes. Each lobe has many smaller 'lobules' which end in tiny grape-like bulbs where milk is produced. 2. Milk ducts – slender tubes that carry the milk from the lobes to the nipple. 3. Fat. 4. Connective tissue.

**Breast care nurse** A specialist nurse who offers support and advice to breast cancer patients.

**Breast-conserving treatment/surgery** Operation to remove the cancer and a small amount of normal breast tissue.

**Breast implant**  Silicone sac filled with saline (salt water) or silicone gel. The sac is placed under the skin behind the chest muscle.

**Breast reconstruction**  A surgical procedure which aims to create a 'new' breast using an implant or tissue. Used in cases where either a whole breast or substantial tissue has been removed.

**Cancer**  The uncontrolled and abnormal growth of cells.

**Cancer Networks**  There are 34 Networks in the UK, with one or two key hospitals in each area which provide a full range of cancer care and treatment.

**Capsular contracture**  This occurs when fibrous scar tissue forms around an implant, making it hard and painful.

**Chemoprevention**  The use of drugs to prevent cancer.

**Chemotherapy**  Treatment with cytotoxic (anti-cancer) drugs.

**Clinical oncologist**  Another name for a radiotherapist who is an expert in giving and planning any radiotherapy.

**'Comfy' (soft prosthesis)**  A light prosthesis made of synthetic washable fibre.

**Consultant**  A physician or surgeon who does not take full responsibility for a patient, but acts in an advisory capacity.

**Cording**  Refers to the raised cord-like strings of fibrous tissue that can develop down the arm or side of the body. It is thought to be the result of clotted or thrombosed lymph vessels. Although not harmful, cording can be uncomfortable and restrict movement.

**Core biopsy**  The removal of a sliver of tissue under local anaesthetic, which is then examined under a microscope to check for abnormalities.

**CT (CAT) scan**  A type of X-ray that takes pictures from different angles. These pictures are put together and form a detailed picture of the inside of the body, enabling the site of a cancer and the extent of its spread to be identified.

**Cyst**  A non-cancerous fluid-filled sac that can develop in the breast tissue.

**Cytological testing**  The removal of a sample of cells for testing.

**DIEP (Deep Inferior Epigastric Perforator)**  A type of breast reconstruction in which skin and fat with its own blood supply is taken from the abdomen to make the breast shape.

**Distant spread**  The recurrence of breast cancer in other parts of the body. Also known as secondary breast cancer.

**DNA**  The molecule that encodes the genetic information in the nucleus of the cells. It determines the structure, function and behaviour of the cells.

**Doppler Ultrasound**  Specialised type of ultrasound scan in which blood flow is shown up as different colours on a monitor. As tumours have an increased blood supply, this helps identify the site and spread of a tumour.

**Drains**  After an operation wound, drains stop blood and tissue fluid collecting around the operation site.

**Ductal Carcinoma In Situ (DCIS)**  Abnormal but non-invasive cells present within the ducts of the breast.

**Excision biopsy**  A surgical procedure to remove a lump under local or general anaesthetic.

**Extended LD flap** Tissue is taken from the large back muscle (the Latissimus Dorsi) and positioned into the envelope of breast skin. The tissue is taken with its own blood supply and is used to reconstruct breasts without using an implant.

**External radiotherapy** A form of radiotherapy in which high-energy X-ray beams are directed at the breast and/or armpits by a radiotherapy machine to kill off any stray cancer cells.

**Family history clinics** Clinics where women who have a family history of breast cancer can be assessed to try to determine what their individual risk is.

**Fat necrosis** The death of fat cells in the breast caused by failure of the blood supply. May result in areas of hard lumps on the reconstructed breast.

**Fibrocystic disease** A non-cancerous breast condition in which multiple cysts or lumpy areas develop in one or both breasts.

**Fibrosis** The build-up of scar tissue.

**Fine needle aspiration** Procedure in which a sample of breast cells is taken using a fine needle. The cells are sent to the laboratory to check for signs of cancer.

**Free TRAM flap** The reconstruction of the breast using tissue which is detached from its existing blood supply and re-connected, using the vessels that come from the upper end of the abdomen and joining them, by microscope, to vessels either from under the breast bone or from the armpit.

**Gene** Genes are formed from DNA, carried on chromosomes and are responsible for the inherited characteristics that distinguish one individual from another. They also govern the structure and functions of the body's cells.

**Gene test** A blood test to check whether a patient's DNA has a faulty gene which might predispose them to cancer.

**General plastic (cosmetic) surgeon** A surgeon who doesn't specialise exclusively in breast reconstruction.

**Genetic mutation** This occurs when some of the genes in the cell are damaged or lost, sometimes causing particular conditions or diseases or a predisposition to certain conditions or diseases.

**Glands** Organs that produce substances needed by the body (such as hormones) and release them through ducts or directly into the bloodstream.

**Haematoma** The accumulation of blood under a wound that can cause swelling, discomfort and hardness.

**HER2** Some breast cancers contain a large amount of the protein HER2. This protein is a growth factor receptor which stimulates the cancer cells to divide.

**Herceptin (trastuzumab)** A drug that stops HER2 stimulating the growth of cancer. It also increases the effect of chemotherapy drugs on breast cancer.

**Hormone (endocrine) therapy** Treatment that blocks the effects of hormones on cancer cells to stop or slow their growth.

**Hormone receptor positive tumour (oestrogen receptor positive ER+ve, progesterone receptor positive tumour PgR+ve)** Some breast cancer cells have hormone receptors. If hormones produced by the glands, or by the tumour itself, latch onto these receptors, this can stimulate the growth of the tumour. Tumours that are oestrogen receptor positive are termed ER+ve.

Tumours that are progesterone positive are known as PgR+ve.

**Hormone receptors** All normal breast cells have receptors for the hormones oestrogen and progesterone. These receptors allow the hormones to act on the breast during the menstrual cycle and during pregnancy.

**Hospice** A place dedicated to providing symptom control, where staff are specially trained in palliative care.

**HRT (hormone replacement therapy)** A treatment used to reduce or eliminate menopausal symptoms. This involves taking synthetic female sex hormones to replace those the ovaries no longer produce after the menopause.

**Immediate reconstruction** Breast reconstruction that is carried out at the same time as a mastectomy or lumpectomy.

**Induced menopause** This occurs when treatment stops the production of oestrogen by the ovaries. Menstruation should start again after the treatment has ended unless the patient has had ovarian ablation, which induces the menopause and is permanent.

**Inflammatory Breast Cancer** A rare but fast-growing type of breast cancer which causes the skin of the breast to feel hot and look red and inflamed. The skin of the breast may also be pitted like the skin of an orange (known as *peau d'orange*). This is caused by cancer cells blocking the channels through which lymph flows in the breast.

**Internal radiotherapy (brachytherapy)** During this treatment radioactive wires are inserted into the breast tissue under general anaesthetic. This allows an extra dose of radiotherapy to be delivered to the area surrounding the tumour. The treatment involves a hospital stay and nursing staff and visitors may be limited to minimise their exposure to radiation. Once the wires are removed, the radioactivity disappears.

**Invasive breast cancer** Cancer that has spread to the surrounding tissue.

**Invasive Ductal Cancer** This is the most common type of breast cancer and is usually noticed as a lump. The cancer arises in the lobule at the last branch of the ductal tree draining the duct (together known as the terminal duct lobular unit).

**Invasive Lobular Cancer** Accounts for around 10% of diagnosed breast cancers and occurs in the cells that line the lobules of the breast. It is most common in women between 45 and 55 years old.

**Klinefelter's syndrome** A rare genetic condition where a man is born with an extra female chromosome, making him XXY instead of XY. Although men with Klinefelter's are about 20 times more likely to get breast cancer than the average man, the overall risk is still very small.

**Latissimus Dorsi** The widest muscle of the back which lies below the shoulder and behind the armpit.

**L-D flap** Breast reconstruction using a portion of skin, fat and muscle usually taken from the large back muscle (Latissimus Dorsi) which is then formed into a breast-shaped mound together with an implant.

**Lightweight prosthesis** An artificial breast made from silicone gel that fits into a bra and weighs less than a normal prosthesis.

**Liver scan** A type of ultrasound scan used to check whether cancer has spread to the liver.

**Lobular Carcinoma In Situ (LCIS)** This means that there are cell changes in the lining of the breast lobules. LCIS is not classified as a cancer as such, but having it means that you have an increased risk of developing future breast cancer.

**Lobules** Glands in the breast that produce and store milk.

**Local anaesthetic** An injection into the tissue which results in a small area of numbness. The patient is conscious for the whole procedure.

**Local recurrence** The recurrence of cancer in the same breast. This may be due to cells left after surgery or the development of a new tumour.

**Local treatment** This is treatment aimed at the breast itself and the axillary lymph nodes. It aims to eradicate the cancer from the area before it spreads. An example of a local treatment is radiotherapy.

**Lumpectomy** Surgery in which only the lump and a small area of surrounding normal tissue is removed.

**Lymph** The colourless fluid that circulates around the body tissues and contains a high number of white blood cells.

**Lymph nodes** These are small, bean-shaped glands located throughout the lymphatic system. The lymph nodes store special cells that can trap cancer cells and bacteria travelling through the body.

**Lymphatic system** A network of vessels that runs throughout the body transporting lymph. The system is part of the body's immune system and helps defend it from infection and disease.

**Lymphocytes** These are white blood cells that fight infection and disease.

**Lymphoedema** This refers to the swelling caused by a build-up of lymph fluid in a part of the body. This build-up can be caused by cancerous cells blocking the ducts and glands through which the lymph fluid would normally flow. Scars from surgery or radiotherapy can also block the lymph ducts.

**Macmillan nurse** A nurse who is specially trained in caring for people with cancer. They specialise in pain and symptom control and can provide counselling and emotional support.

**Magnetic Resonance Imaging (MRI)** A scan that uses magnetism to build up a picture of the inside of the body. Can be used to detect some cancers.

**Malignant** The term used to describe a tumour that is cancerous. The cancer cells are capable of invading and destroying surrounding tissues and forming secondary tumours elsewhere in the body.

**Mammogram** An X-ray of the breasts that is used to detect breast cancer early, when lumps are 2cm in diameter or less in size.

**Mastectomy** An operation to remove the whole breast.

**Medical oncologist** A cancer specialist physician in charge of chemotherapy and often overall treatment planning.

**Metastasis** The process by which cells from a malignant tumour travel from the breast to other parts of the body.

**Microcalcifications** Calcium deposits formed either by rapidly dividing breast cells or the death of breast cells. When clustered in one area, they may indicate the presence of cancerous cells.

**Micrometastases** When only a few cancer cells have spread from the breast.

**Modified radical mastectomy (also called Patey mastectomy)** A mastectomy which removes the breast and lymph nodes under the arm but leaves the chest wall muscles intact.

**Monoclonal antibody** An antibody (substance that causes an immune response in the body) that can be made in the laboratory in large quantities. The monoclonal antibody Herceptin is used in the treatment of breast cancer.

**Multi-disciplinary breast cancer team** A group of different specialists who meet regularly to discuss each person's case and share their expertise.

**Neoadjuvant or primary chemotherapy** Chemotherapy used to shrink a large tumour so that it can be operated on.

**NHS National Screening Programme** The programme provides free breast screening every three years for all women in the UK aged 50 and over.

**NICE ( National Institute for Clinical Excellence)** A Government body set up to overcome what was known as the 'postcode lottery' of cancer treatment. NICE reviews all types of treatment and, if they approve a treatment, Health Authorities are committed to providing it where it is deemed necessary.

**Oestrogen** A female sex hormone produced by the ovaries. It causes the breast cells to divide during the menstrual cycle to prepare the body for a potential pregnancy. However, oestrogen can also stimulate the division of cancer cells.

**Oncological specialist breast surgeon** Specialist in performing mastectomies.

**Oncoplastic surgeon** Surgeon who combines the skills of breast cancer surgery with those of breast reconstruction.

**Oophorectomy** Surgery to remove the ovaries.

**Osteoporosis** Brittle bone disease that can affect postmenopausal women.

**Ovarian ablation** A low dose of radiotherapy is used to switch off the action of the ovaries. The procedure is used for pre-menopausal women with breast cancer to stop the oestrogen supply to a breast tumour.

**Ovulation** The release of an egg from an ovary for fertilisation during a woman's monthly cycle.

**Ovulatory cycles** The monthly cycle of a woman's reproductive system, during which an egg is produced (ovulation). If the egg is not fertilised, the lining of the womb is shed as a period. It takes roughly 28 days to complete the cycle.

**Paclitaxel (Taxol)** A chemotherapy drug which stops cancer cells dividing and therefore blocks the growth of the cancer.

**Paget's Disease** A rare type of breast cancer in which cancer cells travel from the ducts lying beneath the nipple onto the nipple itself, causing a red, scaly rash. There may also be a lump beneath the nipple.

**Palliative care** If a cancer can no longer be actively treated, palliative care is used to help ease its symptoms. The focus of palliative care is on quality of life rather than a cure.

**Palpable** Refers to a tumour or lump that can be felt beneath the skin.

**Partial prosthesis** Either a hollow 'shell' that fits over the remaining breast tissue creating a more rounded shape, or a crescent of silicone that fills the bra.

*Peau d'orange* A French term used to describe skin that becomes ridged or pitted like an orange during Inflammatory Breast Cancer.

**Phyto-oestrogens; plant oestrogens** Weak plant oestrogens that mimic the action of the female sex hormone.

**Pituitary downregulators** A group of drugs that stop oestrogen production temporarily by acting on the pituitary gland. They are only used on pre-menopausal women.

**Pre-cancerous changes** This refers to cell changes within the lining of the breast lobules. It is not cancer but means you have an increased risk of developing breast cancer in the future if these pre-cancerous changes are not treated.

**Progestogens** Synthetic forms of the female sex hormone progesterone.

**Prognosis** A forecast as to the possible outcome of a disease.

**Prophylactic mastectomy** The removal of both breasts in women who have a high risk of developing breast cancer to try to reduce the risk.

**Prosthesis (breast)** Artificial breast worn inside the bra.

**Radical mastectomy** Procedure in which the breast and axillary lymph nodes are removed, together with the chest wall muscles. This operation is rarely performed.

**Radiographer** A technician who takes X-rays.

**Radiologist** A doctor who specialises in the use of X-ray and other scans.

**Radiotherapist** A doctor (sometimes called a clinical oncologist) who is an expert in planning and giving radiotherapy.

**Radiotherapy** Treatment using high-energy rays to kill cancer cells.

**Raloxifene** A drug which blocks the effects of oestrogen.

**Recurrence** The point where cancer cells from a primary tumour are detected following the primary treatment of the cancer.

**Regional recurrence** Cancer that has recurred in the area around the breast.

**Scalp cooling** A patient wears a cooling cap during chemotherapy. That decreases blood flow in the scalp and thus the amount of drug reaching the hair follicles on the head. As a result, the hair is less likely to fall out.

**Secondary breast cancer** The recurrence of breast cancer in other parts of the body.

**Self-supporting prosthesis** A prosthesis that can be stuck onto the skin either directly or using adhesive tape.

**Sentinel Node Biopsy** A method for checking potential spread of cancer to the lymph nodes. It involves injecting a small amount of radioactive liquid around the cancerous area before surgery. A scan is then done of the nodes to see which have taken up the radioactive liquid. At surgery a blue dye is also injected around the cancer and is taken up into the draining lymph channels and moves to the nodes. Only the nodes that are radioactive or blue are removed and checked for cancerous cells.

**Seroma** Refers to the collection of fluid around the wound after drains have been removed. Seroma causes swelling and pain and increases the risk of infection. It usually goes away on its own but can be drained.

**Simple implant (subcutaneous reconstruction)** This is very rarely done. It involves placing an implant just under the skin and fat.

**Stereotactic or Ultrasound Guided Biopsy** The use of ultrasound to guide a biopsy needle to obtain a sample of tissue/cells for analysis.

**Subcutaneous mastectomy** The breast tissue is removed except for the nipple and areola and the bulk is replaced with a prosthesis.

**Submuscular reconstruction** The most common type of reconstruction whereby an implant filled with saline or silicone gel is inserted beneath the muscle of the chest wall to replace the tissue that has been removed.

**Tamoxifen** The most widely used anti-oestrogen drug. It blocks oestrogen receptors within breast cancer cells, thereby preventing them from multiplying.

**Tissue expander** This is an implant similar to a small balloon. It is gradually filled over a period of weeks through a small port to create a pocket under the chest muscle of a size and shape to match the other breast.

**Tissue expansion** A method of stretching the skin of the chest to accommodate an implant.

**Total or simple mastectomy** Procedure to remove all the breast tissue but not the lymph glands.

**TRAM flap (Transverse Rectus Abdominis Muscle)** Skin, fat and muscle are taken from the lower abdomen to create a new breast shape. Synthetic mesh may be used to reinforce the abdomen wall and protect against abdominal hernias. There is a risk of some of the fat and skin dying due to a poor blood supply to the flap tissue.

**Triage system** Surgeons allocate priority to women whose GPs think they need to be seen urgently.

**Tumour** An abnormal mass of tissue that results from excessive and uncontrolled cell division. Tumours may be either benign or malignant.

**Tumour grading** The grading scale usually ranges from 1 to 3. Grade 1 tumours are composed of cells that closely resemble normal ones. Grade 3 tumours contain very abnormal-looking and rapidly growing cancerous cells.

**Tumour markers** These are produced by the tumour or the body in response to the cancer and can often be detected in higher than normal amounts in the bloodstream if a tumour is present.

**Tumour marker tests** The use of tumour markers to determine the nature of cancer cells and how they might respond to treatment.

**Tumour staging** The stage of a cancer describes its size and spread. This will aid in decisions about treatment.

**Ultrasound** A scan using sound waves to build up a picture of the inside of the body.

**Wide local excision** Also referred to as a lumpectomy. This means surgery in which only the lump and a small area of normal surrounding tissue are removed.

# Index of NHS Hospitals

# Index

abdominal hernia 80, 81, 83
abroad, treatment 134-7
acupuncture 124
addresses 259-60
adjuvant treatments 45, 46, 87-102
    biological therapies 98-9
    chemotherapy 87-94
    clinical trials 99-101
    complementary therapies 101-2
    dietary therapies 102
    hormone therapy 94-8
adrenal glands 96
Adriamycin 99
age
    and breast cancer risk 12-13
    and chemotherapy 88
alcohol intake 9, 14-15
American Cancer Society 14
anaemia 91, 92
anastrozole 22
animal fat 14
anthracycline chemotherapy 115
antibiotics 57, 83
antiperspirants 140
anxiety 28-9, 101
appetite gain 97
appetite loss 63
areola
    rash/swelling 24, 40
    and simple implants 77
    subcutaneous mastectomy 49
    surgery 52, 107
aromatase inhibitors 96-7
aromatherapy 51, 93, 102
asymmetry 83
atypical hyperplasia 8
autoimmune problems 83
axillary nodes
    and cancer recurrence 88, 116
    surgery 48, 49, 54-5, 60, 68

bacteria 55, 92
BASO *see* British Association of Surgical
    Oncology
Bego, Marja 70-71
Benefits Agency 131
benefits and grants 130-31
benign breast disease 7, 8, 27
bilateral cancer 17
biological therapies 98-9, 138
biopsies
    benign breast disease 8
    core 30, 33-4, 35, 36, 147
    excision 34, 36
    male breast cancer 10
    procedure 30
    sentinel node 55
    stereotactic (ultrasound guided) 35-6
birth defects 106, 107
blood tests 120
bloodstream 7, 9
blurred vision 96
body scan 56
bone scan 56, 120
bones
    cancer in 50, 116, 117, 120, 121
    and healthy diet 14

bowel cancer 16
brachytherapy *see* radiotherapy, internal
brain 50, 116, 120, 121
BRCA1 breast cancer gene 16, 19
BRCA2 breast cancer gene 16, 19
breast assessment clinics 25
breast awareness 15
Breast Cancer Care vi, 2, 50, 76, 86, 103, 109,
    111, 112, 130
breast cancer teams 40, 45
    multi-disciplinary 41-2, 44, 46, 60
breast care nurses 20, 30, 40, 42, 43, 44, 47-8,
    50-1, 76, 86, 112, 118
breast changes 24
breast clinics 24
    coping with a visit 31
    procedures 27, 30-31
breast disease, benign 8, 27
breast lumps 24, 27, 28, 141
    benign (non-cancerous) 24-5
    core biopsy 34
    doppler ultrasound 33
    excision biopsy 34
    fine needle aspiration 33
    getting bigger 44
    ignoring 29
    and invasive ductal cancer 39
    lumpectomy 5, 20, 36, 37
    mammograms 31
    and Paget's Disease 40
    statistics 15
    ultrasound scan 32
breast screening 5, 23, 134, 140, 147
Breast Specialty Group vi, 6
breast surgeons (surgical oncologists) 5, 42, 60,
    75, 83-4, 147
breast tissue 28, 66
    location of 19
    mammogram 31, 38
    subcutaneous mastectomy 49
    ultrasound scan 32, 33
breast units 5, 23, 86, 148
breastfeeding 9, 95, 107
BUPA-approved breast units 5, 148

calcium 38, 120
cancer
    bowel 16
    colon 106
    colorectal 146
    defined 7
    endometrial 96
    lung 140, 146
    ovarian 16, 17, 106, 121, 146
    pancreatic 16
    prostate 16, 121, 146
    stomach 16
cancer detection rates 5
Cancer Networks 4, 26, 35, 133, 146, 149-50
    data 151-247
Cancer Research Fund 137
Cancer Research UK 137, 140
cancer units 102, 113
CancerBACUP 76, 90, 106, 130
    Cancer Counselling Service 109
capsular contracture 77, 78, 79, 82
care managers 131
carers 126, 127, 129, 131
cells
    analysis 46, 134

fruit 14, 15

genetic inheritance 8, 12, 13, 15, 16-22
    anxiety concerning family history 28
    chemoprevention 19, 22
    and environment 141
    faulty breast cancer genes 17
    genetic testing 17-18
    and prophylactic mastectomy 18, 19
    risk for family members 41, 43
risk patterns 17
Gerson diet 102
glands, enlarged 24
glossary 261-8
grades of cancer 21, 37, 88
Guide to Grants for Individuals in Need, A 131

haematoma 57
hair loss 92, 103, 105
Harvard School of Public Health, USA 9
Haven Trust 76
healing 101
Health Authorities 136
    five-year survival rates by 248-50
Health Boards, five-year survival rates by 248-50
Health Service Commissioner 139
heart, and healthy diet 14
heart disease 14, 65, 76, 96
heart failure 99
heartburn 63
HER-2 receptor positive 67
HER-2 receptors 67, 98
herceptin 98, 134, 135, 138
Hickman line 90
Hippocrates 109-10
Hippocrates wheat grass diet 102
histology 121
Hodgkin's disease 8
home help 127
homeopathic hospitals 102
hormone receptor positive 67, 88, 95
hormone therapy 42, 45, 56, 94-8
    and recurrence 117, 121
hospices 51, 102, 126, 127, 131-2
Hospital Episode Statistics 146, 258
hospitals
    chemotherapy treatment 91
    choice of 4, 26
    complaints 138
    homeopathic 102
    'imaging' department 30
    index of NHS hospitals 269-71
    introduction of National Cancer Plan 142
    length of stay in 52
    major cancer centres 47
    private 44, 251-7
    radiotherapy department 61
hot flushes 94, 96, 97, 98, 108, 109
HRT (hormone replacement therapy) 9, 13-14,
    15, 27, 43, 94-5
    after breast cancer treatment 99
    combined 13
    unopposed 13
human genome 135
hydrocortisone cream 64
hypnosis 93, 124

ibuprofen 67
'imaging' department 30

immune system 14, 55, 98, 110
immunisations 93
Imperial Cancer Research Fund Breast Cancer
    UK 137
Imperial College of Science, Technology and
    Medicine, London 278
implants 20, 36
    see also under reconstruction
'in situ' disease 38-9, 55
infection 56-7, 83, 91, 92, 93
inflammatory breast cancer 12, 37-8, 43, 89
insurers, and payment for treatment 5
Intensive Care Unit 81
intraductal cancer see ductal carcinoma in situ
invasive breast cancer, and in situ cancer 38, 39
invasive ductal cancer 39
invasive lobular cancer 39
inversion of nipple 24
IUDs (intrauterine devices) 108

Japanese women 16

KC62 screening service returns 258
Klinefelter's syndrome 12

L-D (Latissimus Dorsi) flap 74-5, 76, 79-80, 83
    extended 81
La Leche League 107
laundry 127, 131
law centre 131
LCIS see lobular carcinoma in situ
left-handedness 140
LHRH (Lutenising Hormone Releasing
    Hormone) analogues 97
liver 50, 116, 120
liver disease 9
liver scan 120
lobular carcinoma in situ (LCIS) 38
local recurrence 115, 116
local treatments 45
lumpectomy (wide local excision) 5, 20, 36, 37,
    42, 45, 48, 49, 70, 114
    and breastfeeding 107
    and chemotherapy 90
    and local recurrence 116
    pros and cons 54
    and prostheses 85
    and radiotherapy 60
    reasons for 52, 59-60
    scarring 66
lung cancer 140, 146
lungs 99, 116
lymph 40, 55, 59
lymph nodes 20, 27, 36, 37
    local treatments 45
    spread of cancer to 46, 121
    surgery 48, 49, 54-5, 63
    swollen 27, 114
    tests 20, 48
lymphatic system 7, 116, 117
lymphocytes 55
lymphoedema 58-9, 103

Macmillan Cancer Relief 127, 128-9, 131, 259
macrobiotic diet 102
magnetic resonance imaging see MRI
male breast cancer 2, 8-12, 17, 40
malignant (cancerous) tumours 7
mammary ducts, and breastfeeding 9
mammography 22-3, 25, 27, 29, 30, 31-2

Patient Advisory and Liaison Service (PALS) 138
patient groups 48
*peau d'orange* 39, 40, 56
pectoral muscles 49
periods, early start to 8
phyto-oestrogens 15-16
Pill, the 9, 13, 27, 43, 108
pituitary downregulators 97
pituitary gland 97
plant oestrogens 15-16
plastic surgeons 75
PMT 28
positive thinking 109-10
poverty/affluence 142
pre-cancerous cells 20, 39
pre-operative diagnosis rate 147
preconception counselling 107
pregnancy 106-7
private hospitals 44, 148, 251-57
private medical plans 102
private nursing care 127
private treatment 5, 26, 44, 86
progesterone 13, 94, 97
progesterone receptor positive (PR+ve) 95
progestogens 97
prophylactic mastectomy 18, 19
prostate cancer 16, 121, 146
prostheses 47, 49, 50, 85-6, 111
psoriasis 40
psychotherapy 109, 112
ptosis (droop) 77, 78
pulmonary embolism 56

radiation: exposure and cancer risk 8, 9
radical mastectomy 49, 78, 79
radiographer 31, 32, 62, 63
radiologist 32, 65
radiotherapists (clinical oncologists) 42, 60, 136
radiotherapy 5, 45, 48, 50, 53-6, 60-65, 74, 133, 134, 148
   defined 60
   circumstances in which used 60
   coping with 64
   described 62-3
   external 61
   internal 61-2
   and ovarian ablation 98
   and prostheses 86
   and reconstruction 78, 79
   and recurrence 115, 116, 117
   and secondary cancer 121, 123
   side-effects 63, 64-5
   timing of 61
raloxifene 20
reconstruction 42, 47, 52, 53, 72-84, 85, 114
   and breast care nurse 50
   immediate vs delayed 74-5
   potential complications 82-3
   and prophylactic mastectomy 19
   pros and cons 69, 72
   the surgeon 75-6, 147
   types of 76-81
      simple implant (subcutaneous reconstruction) 77
      submuscular 77-8
      tissue expansion 78-9
      using an implant and the body's own tissue (L-D flap) 79-80
      using the body's own tissue alone 80-81

recurrence 114-24, 137
   and breast implants 84
   and chemotherapy 87, 88
   fear of 53, 54
   and hormone therapy 95
   and key workers 50-51
   local 115, 116
   in other parts of the body 116
   and radiotherapy 60
   regional 116-17
   risk of 115
referral by GPs 4, 17, 25, 26
reflexology 102
regional recurrence 116-17
Relate 109
relationship counselling 109
relatives *see* family
relaxation 93, 101, 108, 124
remission 117, 125, 137
reproductive history 27
research 137
rheumatoid arthritis 83
rights 133-9
risk factors 8-9
   and age 12
   daughters 41
   and HRT 13-14
   and the Pill 13
   recurrence 115
   reducing risk 14-15
   treatments 47
Royal Marsden Hospital, London 110

St Bartholomew's Hospital, London 20
saline solution 78
'scalp cooling' 92
scarring 49, 51, 57, 58, 65, 66, 71, 77, 78, 80, 81,82, 86, 114, 121
scleroderma 83
screening interval figure 258
second opinion 42, 44, 76
secondary breast cancer 7, 37, 87, 115, 116, 117-24
   effectiveness of treatment 123
   emotional response 122-3
   factors affecting treatment 121
   pain control 123-4
   signs and symptoms 117
   tests 120
   tumour markers 120-21
seeds in diet 15
self-examination 15, 20, 51, 114, 119
self-help groups 146
sentinel node biopsy 55
seroma 57, 80, 83
sex life 105-6
side-effects 45, 123
   of biological therapies 99
   of chemotherapy 88, 91-3
   and complementary therapies 101
   of hormone therapy 96, 97, 98
   of painkillers 124
   and palliative care 42, 126
   of radiotherapy 54
silicone 78, 79, 83, 85
simple implant 77
simple mastectomy 49
simulator 62
skin
   changes 24, 114

# Dr Foster Q&A

**Vermilion**
LONDON

### What is Dr Foster?

Dr Foster is an independent organisation which measures healthcare standards through ongoing assessments of every major hospital, maternity unit, care home, consultant, dentist and complementary therapist in the UK. Information from Government, hospitals and medical professionals is analysed with the help of leading universities such as Imperial College of Science, Technology and Medicine, Exeter University and City University. An Ethics committee, made up of some of the most distinguished figures in healthcare, ensures accuracy and impartiality. Supported by the Government and leading professional healthcare organisations, Dr Foster brings together world-renowned academics, healthcare experts and media professionals. For updated information go to www.drfoster.co.uk.

### What makes Dr Foster unique?

For the first time ever, an independent body of experts has assessed the UK's health services ranging from hospitals to maternity services, dentists and complementary therapists. Their unique content derives from questionnaires, statistical research and analysis, contributions from industry experts, individual hospitals, the Department of Health and individual GPs and consultants. These outstanding guides give you the public an unprecedented opportunity to find out how and where to get the best possible care and service.

### Dr Foster Guides

Available now:

| | |
|---|---|
| 0091883792 | Dr Foster Good Birth Guide |
| 0091883776 | Dr Foster Good Hospital Guide |
| 0091883784 | Dr Foster Good Complementary Therapist Guide |
| 0091883814 | Dr Foster Fertility Guide |
| 0091883822 | Dr Foster Breast Cancer Guide |

Forthcoming titles:

| | |
|---|---|
| 0091883857 | Dr Foster Good Care Home Guide |
| 0091883806 | Dr Foster Heart Disease Guide |
| 0091883830 | Dr Foster Good Dentist Guide |
| 0091883849 | Dr Foster Good Consultant Guide |

### How can I order more Dr Foster titles?

To order copies of any of these books direct from Vermilion, an imprint of the Random House Group Ltd, call The Book Service credit card hotline on 01206 255800.

The Dr Foster guides are also available from all good booksellers.